Never Go Back

Never GoBack

Conquering Emotional Triggers Leading to Weight Gain and the Yo-Yo Dieting Dilemma

Joseph Christiano, ND, CNC

with Dwight Bain, NCC, CFLM

Never Go Back by Joseph Christiano, ND, CNC

Published by Body Redesigning
P.O. Box 1088
Deland, Florida 32721
www.bodyredesigning.com

Unless otherwise noted, all Scripture quotations are from the Holy Bible, New American Standard Version. Copyright © 1973, 1978, 1984, International Bible Society. Used by permission.

Cover design by Eric Wilbanks
Interior design and production by Cathleen Kwas

Incidents and persons portrayed in this volume are based on fact. Some names and details have been changed and altered to protect the privacy of the individuals to whom they refer. Any similarity between the names and stories of individuals described in this book and individuals known to readers is purely coincidental and not intentional.

Printed in the United States of America
ISBN (13): 978-0-9789485-0-4
ISBN (10) 0-9789485-0-5

Library of Congress Cataloging-in-Publication Data

Christiano, Joseph.
  Never Go Back / Joseph Christiano, ND CNC

  p. cm.

Contents

Section 1:
Attitude—Never Go Back Attitude

Section II:
Emotions—Connecting with Feelings

Section III:
Diet—Instinctive Eating

Section IV:
Exercise—Body Genetics

Preface

Celebrating 25 Years

I AM A FORMER 305-POUND-DOUGHBOY WHO IS CELEBRATING over 25 years of successfully keeping my weight off. Enjoying my success and vibrant lifestyle for all these years, my personal experience and professional expertise flow through the pages of this book as I take you on a journey that leads you to the answer to never regaining weight. My passion is to be a part of the solution to the obesity epidemic our country faces today by approaching weight loss, weight management, and keeping the weight off for life by addressing the whole person.

Never Go Back is like a road map designed for those who have experienced the frustrations of yo-yo dieting and are looking for the answer to their weight gain/loss dilemma.

The National Registry for Weight Loss, in partnership with the University of Colorado, conducted a survey on weight loss and weight gain and have determined that 95% of people who lose weight through dieting eventually put the weight right back on—often ending up heavier then when they started! Why is that? With Americans being bombarded with so many trendy and seemingly convincing diet plans and with the media constantly propping up the image of lean "hard-bodies," you'd think we'd be a buffed nation, but not so! The sad truth is losing weight is just part of the solution to obesity or being overweight—knowing how to keep it off for life has been the missing resolve to the problem—until now!

Not a diet book!

Never Go Back takes you on a journey of self discovery that leads to the real root problems that cause obesity, being overweight, and regaining weight—a journey filled with inspiration and hope for reaching your fullest potential and your "ideal weight and shape!" You will be empowered to keep it for the rest of your life.

Together with professional life coach, Dwight Bain, I will share insights and thought-provoking information you need to overcome the repeated failure of regaining your weight—once and for all. So get ready to embrace a life of vitality and good health and "never go back!"

Acknowledgements

"Doing common things uncommonly well brings success."
—H. J. Heinz

W HILE I EMBRACE EACH HUMAN'S INDIVIDUALITY, I RESIST individualism as a societal norm. The whole of society can only benefit from the concerted effort of caring and unselfish attitudes embraced by everyone.

It is impossible for me to ever expect such a fine work as *Never Go Back* to be a production of one individual's effort, so my gratitude and thanks go to those who rolled up their sleeves to make this work a success:

Lori—my wife for your support, your intuitiveness, your challenges that make me think deeper, your sensitivity to detail, and awareness in direction—but mainly for your loving under-standing and your love as my helpmate.

Dwight Bain—my good friend and esteemed colleague who supplied his invaluable insights, expertise, and gifts to each reader.

John Weis—for your writing, your creative ideas, your editing input, and for making sure you delivered everything you said you would.

Dave Welday—for assembling all the pieces and players together.

Eric Wilbanks—for the untold number of graphic changes, colors, and text options I requested from you.

Ann Summer—for your expertise, sensitivity to the topic, and pleasant spirit. Every good book needs a good "book doctor." Your surgery certainly was a success!

Michele Randall—for giving me those second pair of eyes with creativity.

Cathleen Kwas—for providing the typesetting and layout.

God—Last on this list, but never least! Humankind could never hope for inner peace, contentment, and eternal life without your supreme example of unconditional love and forgiveness!

Introduction

Never Go Back

Conquering Emotional Triggers That Lead to Weight Gain and the Yo-Yo Dieting Dilemma

M Y PASSION FOR WRITING *NEVER GO BACK* STEMS FROM MY own experience of what being overweight really feels like. I know what it feels like from the inside out. From the outside it appears to be all about one's looks or how one feels physically, but to the overweight person there are additional dynamics which are generally found deep inside which involve emotional hidden trigger points. Because of my personal experience I relate to, and sympathize with, the millions of people who are held captive to this dilemma. My life's journey for successfully losing weight and keeping it off has motivated me to help everyone win this battle for life.

The individual who does not have a weight problem may think that the solution to the problem is simply for the overweight person to cut back on their eating. Unfortunately, it is not that simple and is much easier said than done. The resolution to the overweight problem is much more complicated than just a change in one's diet. I recall the physical limitations and discomforts that went hand in hand with my weight problem, which in many instances caused me to make excuses for not going out in public or attending social events. Being overweight made me feel like I was failing myself instead of improving myself. I found myself walking around emotionally wounded inside an oversized body that didn't belong to me. Besides the physical limitations that existed came the issue of my emotions and attitude about myself. Here I was a prisoner in an oversized body without a clue as to where to begin to unravel the mess I had gotten myself into. Even if I had corrected my diet, it would not have made my problem go away. Keeping the weight off would have been an impossibility because of the underlying emotional/eating issues I needed to address. So the first thing I needed to do to achieve freedom from this stronghold on my life was to identify with my emotions.

Within my oversized body existed an internal battle with my emotions caused by a major personal issue in my life. I was trying to manage my emotional pain through eating, but I was not aware of it. This unhealthy method of coping with my emotions sent me down a road to a place I would never intend to travel—unhappiness and discontentment with the way I looked and felt, but more importantly, the way I felt about myself.

Was what I looked like at 305 pounds in the photo the main problem, or was what I saw in that photo of myself the result of something greater going on inside?

Being blind-sided by a photo of myself, my whole world stood still as I became overwhelmed with the shock of seeing my oversized body crash head-on with my emotionally shipwrecked condition. Panicking to get off this road of destruction, two major questions swirled around in my head: *How in the world did I get into this condition, and how in the world am I going to get out of this condition for good?* Little did I know that the road that would lead me to becoming fit would address my emotions, not what I should eat.

I was convinced that my eating habits—which were out of control—led to my overweight condition. They were not my primary problems, but were symptomatic of some underlying emotional root issues. In desperation I searched for those potential root issues by going back to my upbringing as a child to see if there was a generational connection with my emotions and eating and adulthood. My journey back to my past helped me determine there was, in fact, an attitude connection to eating that was directly linked to the emotional dynamics that were behind my potentially self-destructive behavior.

After identifying the link between my dietary practices as a youngster growing up and the effect those practices had on my attitude towards eating as an adult, I could see clearly how I had made food a means for coping with my emotional pains. As a child I was complimented for eating huge amounts of food at one time—maybe an Italian thing. But as an adult dealing with a very stressful period in my life, eating huge amounts of food became natural. Natural because the food made me feel good about myself, so the worse I felt about myself, the more I would eat. As I began to realize there was more to my physical condition than just overeating, I was able to travel confidently down this new road that would not only allow me to lose the weight, but more importantly to prevent me from ever going back to 305 pounds again! The better understanding I had of the complexities of the emotions I was feeling due to my circumstances and how I felt when I ate, the more confident I became. It was all starting to make sense to me. It was as if a light was turned on and I could see a ray of hope rise within my soul.

So, one day at a time, I went one-on-one with the emotional pain and learned to cope with each emotion directly—but this time without trying to eat my way through them. In doing so, I was feeling emotional relief and excitement. I became more aware of how I felt every time I ate. I made myself ask dumb questions (at the time they seemed dumb) while I ate. Questions like: *Am I sad? Am I excited? Am I angry?* This mental/emotional exercise really helped me put things into better perspective. Prior to this point, these two emotional dynamics were nonexistent in my psyche. I had not developed them yet. But as I stayed focused on my purpose, the tasks didn't matter to me because I was headed in the right direction. Over time I grew stronger with this mental/emotional exercise program which has been a huge part of my success. Realizing the impact of resolving my emotions without using food and developing a positive attitude about myself and growing in my own self-worth, I began to know that I was on the right road. I wasn't out of the woods yet, but I was certain I would succeed.

I was initially motivated to lose the weight at that time by my "Kodak moment." The only thing I could think of every time I saw that photo of myself was, "I never, ever want to look like that again." It wasn't just the resemblance of looking like a human whale that was the ticket, but the photo stood as a reminder of how emotional pain from life's circumstances had begun to defeat me and perhaps eventually destroy my life had I not turned it around.

Weight loss was not my immediate success, but it was a by-product. My immediate success was identifying the underlying emotional trigger points that had gotten me into trouble in the first place. Then, by applying simple mental/emotional exercises, I was able to set myself free emotionally. Once my emotional condition improved, my attitude about myself became positive and I knew that the rest was just a matter of staying the course. Losing weight and keeping it off for life had become a matter of implementing those mental/emotional exercises when necessary and making healthy lifestyle changes based on my physical genetic individuality.

Dropping eighty-five pounds in eight months over twenty-five years ago made a dramatic change in my appearance and was also a catalyst for regaining my self-worth and a positive attitude. Keeping the weight off for twenty-five years has been a matter of renewing my mind about the powerful role emotions play and understanding the role my physical genetic individuality plays when it comes to making the right food and exercise protocol for myself. By recognizing my unique genetic differences, I applied smart eating and smart exercising through the years that helped me reach my genetic potential. And from time to time when I need a little help along the way, I have that photo of me weighing 305 nearby. Its meaning has changed over time. It now serves as the turning point from my emotional and physical defeat to my emotional and physical freedom for life.

Losing weight may be your immediate and primary goal, but keeping it off for life will be your greatest challenge. To do so you may very well have to do as I did and be willing to go back in time to that place where those painful emotional experiences occurred to find resolve, freedom, and a new life. The process will give you emotional strength, confidence in yourself, and the freedom to enjoy life to its fullest.

My purpose for being so open and honest is to motivate and encourage you to believe in yourself. You no longer have to remain in, or become a prisoner of, an oversized body with all the negative ramifications. You are a special individual with unique physical genetic potential and a capacity for developing a powerful emotional state of mind. You have plenty of self-worth and a purpose in this world to make a difference. Learn from the insights and protocols in my book and gain the confidence to **Never Go Back**.

Section I: Attitude

Never Go Back Attitude

Obstacles are those frightful things you see when you take your eyes off the goal.

—Henry Ford

Chapter

1

Focus on the Purpose Not the Task

W HEN IT COMES TO MAKING THE RIGHT DECISIONS IN LIFE, reaching your goals, or attaining your fullest potential, the greatest strength you will need to draw upon is your attitude. The correct attitude is the mental staying power that is directly responsible for succeeding at all your endeavors. The wrong attitude will be the cause of your failings. No one has reached their goals, set new records, or stepped out of the box to tread in uncharted waters without implementing this type of attitude that kept them from drawing on their former attitude. This **Never Go Back** attitude is the type of attitude that will carry you when you aren't sure you can go any further, or when everything and everyone has failed you.

The attitude you maintain about yourself generally comes from outside influences—information you have received from others plus your own personal life experiences. The way you perceive things about yourself will determine the outcome of your level of success that you experience. Believing in yourself, realizing you have self-worth, and developing a healthy self-image, will manifest itself in the form of confidence and assertiveness. This kind of **Never Go Back** attitude is imperative for overcoming the relapses you may have experienced in the past, or perhaps the current challenges you are struggling with that are holding you back.

> The way you perceive things about yourself will determine the outcome of your level of success that you experience.

Change comes hard. If you plan to make changes, then you must develop the correct attitude to do so. Your attitude is constantly challenged either from emotional trigger points that are contributing to eating disorders, trying to stop repeating past failures, attempting to keep your weight off, or confronting unresolved emotional issues. Your attitude will be challenged by the feelings of being unloved, lacking self-significance, or not having self-love. Self-love is very powerful. Just by learning to accept yourself as you are and where you are in life will prevent and/or put an end to the potential destructive eating disorders and illnesses that are commonly experienced by those who have an unhealthy perspective of themselves. If you can hold onto the fact that you are loved, valuable, have a unique potential within you, and are not meant to meet someone else's standard of performance, then your horizons of possibilities will expand far from where they are today. When you practice this **Never Go Back** attitude, you will learn to love yourself, believe in yourself, overcome obstacles, push through challenges and "tasks," and be an inspiration to others.

This attitude is a powerful mental attribute that you possess. It has no boundaries or limitations—it just needs to be developed. As you read this section, take time to do some self-inventory and get connected with your feelings about yourself and others and see where you need to make changes to fill the void(s) in your life.

Stay on Your Purpose

Since you have taken the time to read this book you must have a specific interest in some area of your life that you want to learn more about so you can be successful with your weight. Maybe you've made the decision that it's time to lose weight. It may be that you have tried conventional weight loss diets and have failed at them. It could even be that you actually did lose weight, but failed to keep it off. No matter what the answer is, or where the void exists, you know exactly what you want to accomplish. Perhaps achieving the end result is the part you need help with. So let's start by not getting entangled in the details but rather understanding the important lesson to *focus on the purpose not the task.*

In the Attitude section of my life coaching series "Fork in the Road" (see Appendix B for more information), I make a point of stressing to my clients to make *Focus on the purpose not the task* their personal mantra. I recommend that you repeat these words of empowerment when you wake up in the morning, during the day, and before you go to bed at night. Allow your subconscious to be filled with these empowering words over and over, and over time you will develop the mental staying power to push through the tasks necessary for reaching any of your goals.

The "G" Man
Looking past the tasks and to the future

Let me share a personal story to illustrate what I mean by saying, *Focus on the purpose not the task*. At the age of twenty-five, I had tried several different employment opportunities, had been in the military, attended college to pursue a degree in psychology and special education, and had a family of five to feed.

I intuitively changed the career path I originally chose for my future by getting in touch with my innate gift. I chose to be a natural health professional. I had a natural God-given desire to help people be healthier, so the prospect of being involved in natural health was very appealing to me. To make this all happen was another story, and was not that simple. There were several obstacles to deal with, one of which was to relocate to Florida. Because of the obvious attractions like palm trees, miles of sandy beaches, and the fact that Florida was not known for the snowy, ice-cold winters I was familiar with in Buffalo, New York, I thought that's where I wanted to live.

Another obstacle was the cost of relocating to Florida, making a career change, establishing a new career—not to mention everything else involved in making a major life change. Since my employment at the time paid me $200.00 per week, I had plenty of motivation to do what was needed. But, what could I do to overcome this tremendous challenge to move and make my dream come true?

I was employed at a major sanitation company in western New York. I was a sales rep and sold heavy-duty compactors and waste management equipment—those big cardboard compactors you see in the back of the stores in the malls and shopping centers. Shortly after I started with the company, they lost their dealership. I thought I was going to be in the soup line, but instead I was brought in as the operations manager. It was there one evening when my opportunity for relocating and pursuing my career presented itself.

As the guys finished their garbage routes on a usual cold winter day, they would come into the locker room to change and punch their time cards and leave. I noticed most of the guys were anywhere from eighteen years old to my age of twenty-five. But there happened to be one guy who was much older than the rest. In fact, he was fifty-five years old and looked extremely weather-beaten, tired, and weary. His name was Don.

I felt bad for Don. I asked him how he was doing and he replied that he was dead tired. I asked him why he was still on the back of the G-truck throwing garbage everyday when all the other workers were so much younger than he was. He told me that when the owner of the company and he were kids the owner wanted to start a sanitation company and told Don if he would start with him, he would take good care of him. Well, his old friend and owner of this huge sanitation company forgot Don over the years and consequently Don was stuck on the back of a truck with failing hopes of his friend's promise. My next question was, "If you could do it all over again, what would you do?"

He looked at me and said, "If I were thirty years younger (that was my age, by the way) I would start my own garbage company, grow it, and then sell it and move to where the weather is warm."

As he answered my question, a light as clear as daylight came on…I was that thirty-year-old younger guy! At that very moment I made a decision to become one—a G-man!

I knew the business. I learned the ropes but never was on the back of a truck nor ever wanted to be. This huge task that I was about to take on was not at all what my idea of making a career change was about, but instead was a means to get me there. In my mind all I saw were those sandy beaches, beautiful swaying palm tress, no more snowy, ice-cold winters and becoming a natural health professional: my purpose!

Not coming from money nor having a cent to my name I went to my parents to see if they would cosign a loan with me. All I needed was $5,000.00 to purchase a truck. I had already negotiated a pick-up contract with a homeowners' association. Before I had a truck, I established my first account plus a check from them. As I was explaining to my parents my questionable choice of work, they could see my determination, even though they were shocked. They were gracious to help me with the financing, so I was ready to get things rolling. But before the conversation was over my mother said, "Just don't put your name on the truck." Now I could have taken that as an insult, but instead I used it as fuel to help motivate me for my journey ahead. I knew I was in for a long haul, but didn't realize exactly how long or what it would take to build this business with hopes of one day selling it so I could move to Florida and pursue my dreams.

When I urge you to *focus on the purpose not the task* I know from first-hand experience what I am saying because there were plenty of "tasks" for which I hadn't planned.

I recall those frozen winter days when I had to wake up at 4 AM and shovel my way out of the driveway just to get out on the road, and then drive to the yard where my truck was. Once there I had to try to start a frozen truck engine, and if I could without needing a jump start, I could begin my day. After fighting blizzard conditions, climbing snow banks to get to my customers' garbage cans, freezing my fingers off, and not having any flat tires or accidents, I would return home by 12 o'clock at night. Or how about those hot summer days when the garbage smelled so terrible I could vomit? Or the time I dumped a garbage can in the back of the truck and the soupy garbage with maggots splashed back into my face? *Tasks, tasks, tasks!*

As my company grew, so did the hours, workload, and tasks for this G-man. Do you think I was challenged with keeping a **Never Go Back** attitude? Let's face it, I was doing something for four long years I really didn't want to be doing. I could have easily lost focus of my purpose and given up on my dreams and settled for second best, but because I stayed focused on my purpose and not the tasks, I made it.

When the tasks became overwhelming I made myself look at the future and where I was **going** not where I was. By not getting bogged down with the day-to-day tasks, but staying focused, I was able to accomplish more than a twenty-five-year-old rookie entrepreneur with a family of five and not a penny to his name could ever have dreamed of accomplishing. To make a long story short, I pushed through all the tasks of building my business.

Finally, I reached my goal! I sold my business and moved to Florida. Though my goal from the onset seemed a bit bleak and somewhat impossible, it finally became a reality. Today, I own a natural health and fitness company, I am a naturopathic doctor, and I am absolutely enjoying the fruits from a mantra I learned to use many years ago: *focus on the purpose not the task*. So don't tell me you can't do it!

Oh, by the way, after growing my company for fours years with my trucks being seen all over town, my mother said, "Joey, you ought to put your name on the trucks so everyone will know it is you."

Commitment

When it comes to the mysteries of how to lose weight and keep it off for life, it seems the obvious has been overlooked for many years. We all have a tendency to address the symptoms rather than the root issues when it comes to mastering weight loss for life. With the exception of one's genetics and emotional trigger issues, generally all of us share the same components that are

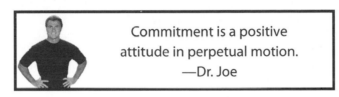

Commitment is a positive attitude in perpetual motion.
—Dr. Joe

necessary to accomplish our weight loss success. Keeping two things in mind, you will get the picture of what is necessary to lose weight and keep it off and will help you to better understand commitment.

The two main components necessary for losing weight are **eating** and **physical activity**. By making these a daily part of your lifestyle, you will increase your metabolism. Your metabolism is key for burning calories. As you know, excess stored calories hide in the form of fat. So if you wish to lose fat then make sure you are continually doing these two things: eating and staying physically active. If you do, then you will create what I refer to as *metabolic momentum*. Metabolic momentum is getting your metabolism up and running and in perpetual motion. As long as you keep your metabolism in perpetual motion, you will not have a problem with your weight until you change one or both of these two components negatively. The difference for success is where your genetics and emotions come into play, but I will address that later in the book. But the point is that in order to reach your weight loss/management goals, you must keep your metabolism in perpetual motion.

Likewise from the mental/emotional side, you must keep your attitude in perpetual motion in order to accomplish your goals—that is what commitment is. To obtain my dreams as a twenty-five-year-old man it was imperative that I *focus on the purpose and not the tasks* and make that mind-set a mental reality so I could stay committed. Commitment has all the possibilities for producing success **if** you know exactly to what you are committed. Did I need to stay committed to my business? No. My future dreams? No. **I had to stay committed to myself.** The journey I choose was for me. It was about accomplishing what I wanted. It wasn't about my family or making money, though they all factor into the big picture—it was about committing to my desire to be all I can and wanted to be.

As you may have experienced in the past, and as you pursue keeping your weight off for life from this day forward, you're probably going to have to deal with your own negative thoughts that arise in addition to running into non-supportive people. You will have personal issues that will come along that could derail you if you let up. This time will be different if you learn to *focus on the purpose not the task*. If you do, you won't give up and go back should you have the occasional bad day. Your confidence won't be shaken to the point that you give up when you hit a plateau. Staying focused means staying committed, but committed to you and you alone. Millions of well-intentioned people have started down the right road only to detour off within a few months because they lost focus of their purpose.

Have you ever watched the Kentucky Derby or other famous horse races on television? If so, you have probably noticed the "blinders" on the outside of each horse's eyes. The purpose of these blinders is to prevent the horse from being distracted by anything that comes into view on either side of his head. The horse's owner and trainers realize how important it is to keep the animal focused. The same is true here.

Don't let any distractions keep you from achieving what you want to get out of life. Dream your dreams, set your goals, and go after that which is valuable to you with a passion. Keep the blinders on!

— Renewing Your Mind —

() Do you find it difficult to finish or complete a task or goal? Yes, or no? If yes, you may want to re-adjust your sights on your target. Many times goals or aspirations in life come slowly. In the process our vision can get a bit blurred, and consequently we lose focus of the intended target. If that is the case for you, consider repeating my mantra—*focus on the purpose not the task.* It may sound ridiculous, but when you are in the middle of the tasks, a little positive affirmation can go a long way. Remind yourself why you are pursuing your goals.

( ) Are you willing to do what it takes to accomplish your long-term goals? Yes, or no? If yes, then keep in mind that losing weight and keeping it off comes in two phases. First, the weight loss phase. Then after the weight is down to an ideal range, keeping it off is long term. My becoming a naturopathic doctor took me on a journey to uncharted waters. Just as each task was a mere stepping stone for accomplishing my goal, you must be willing to take the road that leads you to your destination. Keep your eyes on your destiny, your goal, or your dream, and never go back to where you started.

( ) Many of us can get very excited and even motivated to make changes, especially after being pumped up by someone's success story. But once we jump into the water and find out how cold it is we swim to the side to get out as fast as we can. Do you struggle with the desire and feelings you had about pursuing a goal once you begin? Yes, or no? If yes, then reinforce your thoughts about the causes or reasons you choose that particular venture. A lifelong marriage needs commitment to be successful, and so does everything you set out to do. Spending time with people who will encourage you, support you, and make you accountable will help you stay committed to the goal. It might be your spouse, a good friend, or a workout partner. These are the people who believe in you. Remember your purpose.

A winner is someone who recognizes his God-given talents, works his tail off to develop them into skills, and uses these skills to accomplish his goals.

—Larry Bird

Chapter

2

I Care, Because I am Worth It!

I BELIEVE WHOLEHEARTEDLY IN DEVELOPING THE RIGHT attitude—a positive one—regardless of your endeavors. Perhaps you are planning on losing weight, or you already have but are concerned about relapsing. Or maybe you are making the weight loss, health, and fitness journey for the first time. To do so at this point and time in your life you must be adamant about changing your attitude. It is imperative to examine your mind from time to time to see if you are victimizing yourself by negativity that you have been accustomed to carrying around with you. If you plan to succeed over the course of your life in obtaining your goal(s) you must dump the negative attitude to get there. Only you can do this…and you do have the power.

You may say that you are not a negative person so that won't be a problem for you. I hope that is the case. I realize none of us wants to be classified as a negative person. Still, we have all had plenty of negativity dumped into our minds in the form of negative directives and negative words at some time in our past. In many cases, we are still receiving negativity from others. For example, if your plan is to lose weight and keep it off until you die, I promise you it will be a challenge just to focus on the purpose not the tasks, not to mention dealing with the negative hurdles that come along the way. Some of these hurdles will be emotional trigger points that can cause you to relapse, or just feeling discouraged from not seeing results fast enough. Encountering hurdles along the journey is normal, but if you haven't developed the right attitude they will become roadblocks.

Since your formative years, negative input has been poured into your subconscious mind. Whether from your caretakers, family members, or friends you have been introduced to negativity more than you may realize. Think back and see if you can remember the negative clichés or words used. Do you remember hearing directives with negative words like: *Don't touch that; Don't go there; No you can't; Don't forget; Who do you think you are; You're lazy; You'll never amount to anything; You're not smart enough; You're not thin enough; You're fat; You're sloppy; You're stupid; You're useless, etc.*?

Did you realize that all of that negative input went directly into your subconscious mind and remains there to influence your attitude today when you are faced with challenges in life? You may or may not remember those negative words or directives that your caretakers said to you, but they are recorded for life in your subconscious and are as fresh and alive as if they had just been said to you today. And, if you don't have enough positive input and affirmations in your subconscious to offset the negatives, guess what your immediate attitude will be when you are challenged in life? You know the adage: *Garbage in, garbage out*.

Think back for a moment and try to remember the first major challenge you faced in life whether it was of business nature, personal goal, career move, weight loss, or perhaps the one you are facing right at this moment. What was your mind saying to you when you faced your Goliath? Was it saying *Yes—go for it*! *I can do this,* or was it saying *No way, run away. I could never do that*? Chances are you listened to the **no** voice in your psyche. That's the voice that seems to have the loudest volume, especially when it comes to facing confrontations and challenges and comes from the subconscious mind. It contributes to your being intimidated by others or backing down from opportunities, it interferes with your being stretched so you can reach your potential or causes you to quit before you reach your goals, and it can set you up for failure before you begin. It contributes to low self-esteem and will keep you from being all you can be if you allow yourself to be guided by that negative voice.

What happens when you are guided by the **no** voice is that you develop a defeatist attitude. If you find it difficult to admit you have been courting a negative attitude, your failure rate for success is greater. Like living in denial, not facing the fact that you have a negative attitude may lead to your choosing an unhealthy coping method. You back down by telling yourself the goal or challenge you once planned on accomplishing is not all that important anyway. Consequently you lie to yourself, the hopes you once had are fleeting, and in the end you loose.

Perhaps without even being aware of it, you have been influenced to some degree by those negatives that have been poured into your subconscious mind and now you need to make a little attitude adjustment. So instead of washing your hands and evading the challenges and opportunities in your life that are there for the taking, why not be willing to open your mind and be willing to change? Once you can identify with (or admit) the fact that you need an attitude adjustment, you will be ready to receive positive input and affirmations to offset the negative stuff in your subconscious and create a healthy attitude.

Dumping the *I Don't Care* Attitude

In September 2004, I had the opportunity to implement my *Dump the Junk* after-school health and fitness program at Amos Alfonso Stagg High School in Stockton, California. My curriculum was geared for junior and senior high school students and consisted of three key components: attitude, diet, and exercise. The students who participated in the twelve-week program volunteered and were classified as obese and at-risk kids. At-risk means the students had failing grades, poor attendance records, poor classroom participation, and overall less than desirable attitudes. Some came from broken homes. Some were physically abused, some emotionally abused, some sexually abused, some were living with sponsors or relatives, and some were involved in gangs, etc.

The students went through physical fitness evaluations and tests and were measured for body compositions, BMI, body fat, and lean muscle weight. The findings showed that the majority were either overweight or obese, so you can imagine the challenge I was facing. It was a classic example of how an individual's physical condition directly correlates to their mental condition, which in this case, directly affected their academics. For me to help these kids successfully reach their fullest potential in physical fitness and academics, I needed to coach them in developing the correct attitude. I refer to it as addressing the "whole" child.

When I initially visited the school and walked the campus I got a bird's-eye view of what the students were experiencing during lunch period. Of the near 3,500 students, I saw approximately 250 jammed in the cafeteria, several hundred eating junk food from the vendors on the campus, some leaving the campus to go to the local fast-food restaurants, and the remaining thousand or so ate nothing. I was overwhelmed with the dietary problems they faced. It was easy to see how the students' attitudes were a problem. Most of them were undernourished, experienced low blood sugar, and consequently were doing poorly in school because they couldn't stay awake in the classroom or stay focused on the subjects being taught by their teachers. Their home environments, poor dietary practices, and unfit conditions, particularly as teens, had psychological and physiological effects on their attitudes.

After observing the lunch period catastrophe and then interviewing each student, I was filled with compassion to step in and see if I could help these kids. I decided to volunteer my time. I took four months out of my schedule and temporarily moved out to northern California to work with the students personally. I became their fitness trainer, life coach, and friend. It was a wonderful experience, though at times very heartbreaking. My purpose for implementing my program was to establish data that would support my theory that if a student lost weight, improved their physical condition, and learned basic principles of setting boundaries and applying self-control, they would in turn improve their academics.

After twelve weeks, all the students showed tremendous physical improvements including a major reduction in body-fat percentages, lower BMI readings, improved body composition (less fat and more lean weight), loss of weight, and overall improved physical fitness. But the thing that pleased me the most, considering these kids had been labeled as being at-risk, was their newly improved self-esteem, self-worth, and positive attitudes.

When I first met with the students not one of them would look me straight in the eye when I addressed them. They walked around with their heads hung down and when I asked them questions about themselves, their future plans, etc., they just seemed to drift out into space somewhere with no apparent thought or hope for tomorrow. For the most part, they had an *I Don't Care* attitude. I believe their negative attitude came mostly from years of having negative input being dumped into their subconscious minds by their caretakers and the dysfunctional family relationships and environments at home. I doubt very much if any of them didn't want to have a good life with hopes of building a bright future. They developed negative attitudes being victims of their circumstances. No one let them know how valuable they were, or that there was a plan and purpose for their lives. I could tell nobody had taken the time or patience to show them where their negative attitudes had gotten them in their lives and what they looked like having that kind of attitude. In my curriculum there was a list like the one below that helped opened their eyes to see how a *I Don't Care* attitude affected the way they thought about themselves and, in turn, how it affected their decisions.

I Don't Care Attitude Says:

- I don't think very much of myself.
- I don't deserve anything good in life.
- I'm just not smart enough.
- I do not deserve to be healthy.
- I let others treat me with disrespect because I don't respect myself.
- I accept being a loser in life.

For twelve weeks, they spent five days a week in both group fitness classes and a teaching classroom environment. They learned about nutrition and the benefits of exercise. Through repetition (and application of it) they were also experiencing personal growth by being taught and learning to apply the principles of setting boundaries and using self-control. Once they truly felt that someone cared for them and believed in them, they realized they had value. As they accepted the fact that they had value and worth, their self-image improved as did their confidence in themselves. From there I could see them beginning to change emotionally. Some of these teenage girls had scars and cuts on their arms and shoulders from self-mutilation. These scars were outward manifestations of the emotional pain and hurt they had been holding onto since their childhoods. Some of these young people had experienced sexual and physical abuse. They lacked positive words of affirmation to build on. When I saw their state of mind, from time to time I would give them a hug and tell them that I loved them and God loved them. I could tell they didn't know how to handle that kind of talk or affection. I'm sure at first they thought I was weird, but they received the affirmations.

As their belief in themselves grew, so did their self-esteem. These former students who once walked around with their heads hung down when I addressed them with no thought for a bright future, all of a sudden began talking about improving their grades so they could go to college or start their own businesses. These were the kids who had nothing going for them because they were mentally, emotionally, and physically beaten down all their lives. They had had an *I Don't Care* attitude. All of them made a 180-degree turnaround as they were shown how to shut off that **no** voice and turn on the **yes** voice. By learning what was important in their lives like studying for exams instead of going out with their friends, they could improve their academics and graduate. Or, knowing they had value and worth, they set boundaries to protect themselves from intruders instead of remaining in abusive relationships or being a doormat. Or, they realized that by working hard at their goals and staying focused on their purpose, they could be whatever they dreamed they could be. Or, they took time to think first, before picking up a cigarette, using alcohol, drugs, or having sex. As they learned what was important for them, they started establishing standards. From there they could shut off the **no** voice and turned on the **yes** voice. In a very short period of time they were able to set priorities in their lives and strive to become successful.

They went from an *I Don't Care* attitude to an *I Care* attitude about themselves. They experienced their accomplishments in physical fitness by learning how to make themselves work and they saw their grades improve by making smart choices like studying for exams instead of partying with their friends. They all radiated a new attitude about themselves. They learned that they had the power within themselves to choose which voice they listened to regardless of what they were facing. In their curriculum I listed positive affirmations that they were asked to repeat to themselves on a daily basis when facing those negative thoughts or experiencing feelings of doubt or insignificance.

These affirmations are listed below to help you to renew your mind with positive affirmations when it comes to challenges in your life. The result is an *I Care* attitude.

I Care Attitude Says:

▸ I believe in myself.

▸ I care about myself.

▸ I respect myself.

▸ I deserve the best in life.

▸ I am worth taking care of myself.

▸ I am a winner by choice.

Ironically, these formerly obese and at-risk kids became students of positive thinking. For their efforts, their academics improved, they began passing their exams, and their overall GPA's grew by two grades. This is after failing the entire year before. They improved their health and fitness profiles and were no longer the former obese or overweight kids. They believed in themselves, which opened their minds to the reality that they had the power within to accomplish anything they chose when they put their minds to it. They learned the value and importance of setting boundaries, applying self-control, and chose no longer to own an *I Don't Care* attitude.

Will You Be a Volunteer?

I had been counseling a gentleman about the concerns he had about his health, his weight, and how he was feeling in general. He said he loved to eat, was a smoker, and was overwhelmed by his work schedule. But he was ready to make a commitment to whatever it took to get his health in order and lose all the weight he had gained over the years. He said he was fifty years old, but he felt like a seventy-year-old man and could feel the downward spiral as his youth left him. He continued to explain that he was on medications for high cholesterol, high blood pressure, his breathing was becoming more difficult, and he was feeling tired all the time.

I discussed all the aspects of what I felt he was going to need to do. To improve his current health status he needed to consider his genetic individuality, how certain foods would be best for his chemistry, exercises to match his body genetics, plus develop a **Never Go Back** attitude. I reiterated that he needed to adopt a mental attitude that this would be a lifetime commitment, not a ninety-day makeover. I could tell by the questions he posed and the look in his eyes that he was thinking more about all the *tasks* to get there and not about his purpose. So to better help him *focus on the purpose and not the task,* I suggested that he take the time to evaluate the importance of making these lifestyle changes. How important was this to him? I explained to him that everyone who makes healthy lifestyle changes is motivated by something unique to their person—this is where one's individuality comes into play. Generally most people make a decision to lose weight because of an event. Event-driven motivation is good to a degree but is very shortsighted. Usually it is a wedding, graduation, reunion, or some event that drives people to get in shape. The individual works diligently at being very careful of what they eat, they make sure they exercise regularly and stay focused on their purpose or goal—the event! But after the event is over and all the compliments have sizzled out, the desire to stay the course dwindles to nothing and over time (a short time at that) they regain their original weight they carried before the event. So if he wasn't careful, the same would happen to this gentleman.

I went on to say that there are usually two primary motivational factors that help people decide to make healthy lifestyle changes. Either we change because we see the writing on the wall and volunteer (so to speak) to do something about it, or we are forced into it because our health is turned upside down, at which time everything we had going on came to a screeching halt.

As I ended our session I left him with this question: which is it for you? Do you want to volunteer, or do you want to wait until you have to make the changes? After a few weeks had gone by he stopped by to say he was too busy at this time to start. Unfortunately, he remains a walking time bomb looking for a place to go off.

How about you? Aren't you worth it? Will you volunteer to make changes, or will you be forced to?

Missing the Point

A woman once came to me with many health issues coupled with the fact that she was overweight. She played all of that down. She was a professional, worked at a desk, and attended meetings, but for the most part her work life was void of physical activities. Her personal life was sedentary, also. She was in her mid-forties and had a poor attitude about exercise and fitness but here she was, sitting at my desk and wanting to find her long lost youthful figure again.

We met three times a week. I was subtly advancing her workout intensity so she would burn more calories and improve her cardiovascular condition. I knew to move her physically within the limits of her current condition, but it was her mental condition that needed the greatest help. I helped her with her food selections and what to do when we weren't training together, and I kept motivating her with positive affirmations. But every day we met, her attitude remained as negative as it could be. She always complained, didn't like her results, and she hated sweating. Absolutely nothing was going to convince her that this personal trainer and his healthy mind-set and protocol for developing a healthy body would make her stay with it. In less than two months she quit.

A month or so later I happened to run into her one day as she and her husband were walking together. As we caught up to each other she grabbed her husband's arm and said, "See I have a husband, I don't need to worry about how I look." What she didn't see is what I saw, and that was the look on her husband's face. Here was this woman beaming with a smile like the cat who just ate a bird, and her husband looked totally dejected and insignificant.

I am not telling you this story in order for you to feel it necessary to get into shape for your spouse's sake, but I am sharing this with you so you will realize that making healthy lifestyle changes will affect **every** aspect of your life. Everyone is unique. It's our individuality that drives our motivation. Don't be shortsighted or event-driven to lose weight. Events can become the catalyst for reaching long-term goals, but develop and keep the mind-set to make your weight problem and health a priority whether there is an event or not. Every area of your life will be positively influenced when you are in good shape. Don't let poor health be the motivational factor, either. Be a volunteer. Receive the benefits for life.

So as you prepare to step out and go for the gold let me help you better prepare by asking you: *How important is it for you lose weight and keep it off until you die? To improve your illness profile and enjoy a vibrant, energetic, and disease-free life?* The level of importance will be the determining factor as to the outcome of your journey.

Why Bother?

Some years ago when I was involved in personal training, I had a female client whom I had been training for over a year. We had developed a wonderful relationship and we got to know each other pretty well. During one of our sessions she had asked me what I did personally to stay in shape. It's always funny to me when someone asks me that question because it really makes me think about what I do, probably because staying in shape is such a normal part of my life. Being a normal part of my lifestyle I don't really look at it as something I **have** to do but rather something I **choose** to do and I just do it. I explained to her my exercise regimen was based on my body genetics and the type of exercises I preferred were based on instinct rather than on following a certain program. And how often I exercised per week and the intensity of my workouts were based on my energy level. Then I told her about my preferred choice of eating and that I didn't believe in dieting but believed to be as accurate as I could in making food selections that would be compatible to my blood type. And, of course, taking dietary supplements. (Please see Appendix A for a complete list of supplements and products.) In her amazement she responded, "You are going to have to do that for the rest of your life?"

I nearly fell to the floor laughing. I was taken by surprise by her comment. Here I was, making a healthy lifestyle my practice since I was a teen, and she thought I would have to keep doing it! *Was there another way*, I thought to myself?

My attitude about taking care of my body and staying in shape has everything to do with what is important to me. In my competitive days it was about being rock hard, muscular, defined and symmetrical and willing to walk out on a stage in front of hundreds of people in a Speedo. As I age, my motives or reasons why I bother are different. I don't care to be a part of the competitive scene anymore (and certainly the Speedo thing) but I do care about the many benefits I receive from staying in shape. I thrive on the mental side of it. It gives me a real sense of accomplishment. I enjoy feeling energetic. I very seldom get a cold or sick. I like being physically active. A clear mind, regular exercise, making food selections for my blood type, taking supplements, thinking positively, and growing in faith in God all enrich my life. Why stop now? I enjoy life and the many things that are priceless in my life like my wife, my children, my grandchildren, friends, and business. These are all motivational factors that make it all worthwhile for me to stay in shape so I can enjoy them to the fullest. I am not interested in trying to look younger or even act younger. I could not imagine being caught up in a mind-set of wishing that I could be like I was when I was thirty years old. I like my life right now, right where it is. I see staying in shape and maintaining a healthy lifestyle as a necessary component because of the positive effects it has in every aspect of my life. Unlike my gentleman client who knew he needed to turn his unhealthy condition around but discovered it wasn't important enough for him to change. He didn't see the positive impact it would have on his personal life and others in his life.

I cannot make you decide to do the things it takes to get your weight down to where it needs to be and your body and health in shape. You have to decide to do this on your own with the benefit of whatever assistance I can offer you. As you are learning to make the proper attitude changes, you also need to apply that attitude when it comes to setting your goals. Goals generally stem from what motivates you most. They have to be of value and of importance to develop the **Never Go Back** attitude.

Let me give you some things to think about, but your motivational reasons are personal and are yours only. Those reasons you list are why you should bother.

Goals with Value

Setting goals is easy. Reaching them is an entirely different story. It will be their level of importance to you that will make it possible for you to attain them. Your goals may involve a loved one like your spouse, children, career, occupation, health, longevity, spirituality, etc. The following are a few ideas you might want to consider before writing your goals down:

- ▶ *Your goals should have value.* They are yours and belong to you and no one else, but make them your personal possessions. Treat them as if they were sacred treasures. If they are not valuable to you, how do you think you will possibly find the energy and ambition to bother with them for life? Treat them as valuable. Remember: the level of importance that you apply to them will determine the outcome.

- ▶ *Put a price tag on your goals.* That's how valuable they should be to you. For example, how much value is there in reaching your weight loss goal? Tag it. Is it worth $10.00? $1000.00? Or $1,000.000? It must have a value or you will not find the physical and mental energy to successfully attain it.

- ▶ *Write your goals down where they can be seen.* You need the constant reminder of what they are, so be certain you write them on something that is easily visible. For example, place your list of goals on the refrigerator door, your desk at work, in your wallet, in the bathroom—wherever you need for them to be so you can see them often. By revisiting your list of goals on a day-to-day basis you will be re-enforcing your mind in a way to stay *focused on the purpose not the task.*

▶ *Speak your goals out loud.* By verbalizing your goals you are telling yourself what is on your heart. And what is on your heart is what you are and what you believe. This is a very powerful method for becoming successful because you are reminding your mind of what you want to be or accomplish while re-enforcing your mind that you will be it or, in the case of setting a goal, reach it.

▶ *Your goals should be both short term and long term.* An example of a short-term goal is losing weight. Keeping your weight off is an example of a long-term goal. Setting short-term goals is a positive method of building self-confidence while you are pursuing your long-term goal. Short-term goals provide mental and physical rewards more frequently and offer constant feelings of accomplishment.

▶ *Be specific about your goals.* They should not be fuzzy or generalities. Your goals need to be specific, or you will hit the wrong goal. Your goals need to be clear. For example, don't say you would like to weigh around 165 pounds some day. That is too general. Your goal is to weigh 165 pounds. So set your sights for weighing in at 165 pounds. That is a specific and clear-cut goal.

▸ Include a friend to hold you accountable when you are setting your goals. Being held accountable is a powerful dynamic for success. This person must be positive and open-minded. They must be honest enough to let you know when you are slipping or relapsing. This is the person you want to cover your back. There should be an element of trust between you that is dependable and reliable.

Attitude is the cornerstone of failure or success, depending upon what attitude you choose to embrace. Having been bombarded with more negativity in your life then you will ever need, now is the perfect time to adhere to the positive side of your mind—the **yes** voice. Take time to think through what I have written above and throughout this section of the book on attitude. The mental exercises are key for building the mind for success.

Remember the saying: "Sticks and stones may break my bones but words will never hurt me?" How far from the truth was that line when we were kids? Sure those sticks and stones may breaks bones, but man those words or (name-calling) definitely hurt. It is called emotional pain. Don't allow the negative experiences in your past to influence your choices for today. If you need to forgive an individual who caused you emotional pain, then do it so you can be free. Don't remain under the influence of the **no** voice any longer. Chapter Four will help you to discover how to avoid the **no** voice even more.

Your subconscious mind is like a vault that holds the good and the evil—the negative and the positive, but it will depend on which voice you listen to the most. Choose today which voice you will listen to and enjoy the freedom of overcoming negative thoughts. Fill your mind with good, honest, pure, and positive thoughts about yourself and others.

As you make your life the life it was destined for by reinforcing your mind with the positive goals and purposes you have selected, you will find it easy and fulfilling to dump the negative attitude.

— Renewing Your Mind —

You don't have to be affected by negative people who have negative things to say to you anymore.

() Negative people will influence your attitude in a negative way. Positive people will influence you in a positive way. Do you make it a habit of surrounding yourself with negative people? Yes, or no? If yes, then do your best to avoid them or minimize your time with these people. Do not bother sharing your goals or aspirations with them. They will not see past their pessimistic attitudes. Seek out positive people who are successful, driven to excellence, and optimistic. Positive people will encourage you with your dreams and goals and are open to change.

() Losing weight is easy; keeping it off for life is a different story. Have you ever tried to lose weight but couldn't keep it off? Yes, or no? If yes, then developing the **Never Go Back** attitude is the place to begin. This attitude teaches you how to refuse to repeat the things that made you fail in the past. To make that attitude a daily part of your life, be a constant positive thinker. Focus on your purpose and reinforce yourself with affirmations like: *I believe in myself; I have value and worth; I choose to be a winner in life; I will succeed!* Also review Goals with Value to remind yourself of how important your goals are to you. It won't be long before you will refuse to own any negative feelings about yourself. You will no longer be stopped from being all you can be.

*I count him braver who over-
comes his desires than him who
conquers his enemies; for the
hardest victory is over self.*

—Aristotle (Greek Philosopher)

Chapter

3

Self-control and Setting Boundaries

BOUNDARIES AND SELF-CONTROL ARE YOUR COMBAT twins, or the powers within, that are at your disposal. They are not intended to restrict you from becoming everything you ever wanted to become or to prevent you from reaching your wildest dreams, but rather to assist you in becoming everything you ever wanted to be.

Combat Twins for Protection

Setting boundaries and applying self-control are two very powerful actions you can use to protect yourself from a myriad of negative assailants, both from within and without. Whether you deal with overindulgence, uncontrolled desires, impulsive decision making habits, backsliding into former habits that cause failure, an abusive relationship, never learning to set boundaries as a child and today are struggling with eating disorders, or poor self-esteem, there is hope.

When you want to pull off this road that leads to losing weight and keeping it off forever, then just think about some methods of applying self-control. Who in the world wants to apply self-control when it comes to making food selections, especially when those emotions kick in and you need to medicate? Self-control probably means no more *Little Debbies*. Or how about whether you should exercise or not? And if so, how much, when, and where? Forget about it! Self-control reminds most people of restrictions and limitations…plus, who has ever really been taught how to put on the brakes?

In Chapter One you learned why it is important to *focus on the purpose not the task* and why it should become your daily mantra. Well, now your journey for being successful is going to require a couple tasks. So instead of taking the next exit ramp off this road and avoiding the task of applying self-control, please stay the course and continue reading. In this chapter you will get a better understanding of the power within you and the self protection you need to make your journey safe and successful.

Self-Control
Protecting Me from Myself!

I was in Okinawa while in the military. Because I was on an eighteen-month tour, I was able to learn quite a bit about the customs of the people and the country as a whole. One thing I gravitated to was martial arts, karate. I was intrigued with Isshin Ryu karate, an Okinawan form of self-defense, so I thought I would see what it was all about. When deciding whether to join the dojo (gym) I met with the sensei (instructor). His name was Frank. He took time to explain the history and concept of this form of karate but told me it wasn't so much about taking out the aggressor, but was about learning how to develop the power within—the power of self-control. That concept didn't come easy for me to learn once I enrolled because all I experienced was being slammed, punched, kicked and beat up on during my martial arts classes. I saw this whole karate thing as a means of learning how to protect myself from my invaders by learning how to physically dismantle them—by protecting my borders. In reality it was much, much more than that.

Had someone told me that I had the power within me to control a flight or fight response from an adrenaline rush when someone was attacking me, I would have never believed him. Or maybe that undiscovered mystery was innately the very thing that intrigued me to participate in the first place. I had the makings of what an athlete needs for becoming great in sports or athletics, so exchanging blow for blow with an assailant to protect myself was common sense thinking for me. It wasn't long after getting my shinbones kicked several hundred times during those early months of conditioning in that dojo that the mental side of this Oriental self-defense training experience started to take hold.

As I learned movements both for offense and defense, I was also learning mental lessons at the same time. What I was learning mentally became the larger part of the picture. As I developed more speed and improved my reaction time, my confidence grew. Just the feeling of knowing I actually knew what to do and how to do it when it came to hand-to-hand combat made the whole experience very gratifying. I was developing my ability to move gracefully and with accurate precision, but my ability to apply self-control actually became more of a confidence builder than my physical abilities. All the lessons and repetitions I went through to earn my belts played a vital role in my ability to learn how to develop and apply self-control. Through repetition I learned not only how to concentrate and focus, but also how to isolate. I learned to improve my reactions and responses to my assailants, not like a street fighter but a martial arts expert. I learned how to apply this *power within* to keep them under control. The old way to duke it out was replaced by this new self-governing power to stay in control so I could maximize my counterattacks and minimize any injuries.

> ...my ability to apply self-control actually became more of a confidence builder than my physical abilities.

Your power to apply self-control will serve as your personal bodyguard, protecting you from yourself. It won't matter what or who your assailant is: whether it is overcoming emotional eating, overeating, overspending what your budget allows, or changing your attitude about your self-worth, having self-control puts you in the driver seat so you can reach your destiny. It is the self-governing power you have at your disposal to protect yourself from every decision you make. **Do not turn off this road.**

Self-control in Life
The power to do the things you ought to do

It always fascinates me how the laws for our highways in America come about. I am certain you have read or heard of the increasing rates of high-speed automobile accidents that occur on the highways of America today. In most cases these high-speed accidents are fatal. So to approach the problem you will see a myriad of strategies applied. For example, the auto makers design automobiles with front, rear, and side air bags, more structural support, and even roll bars. The highway patrol sets their speed traps and radar tripods in efforts to control the speeders. The lawmakers change the speed limits at various points on the highways to prevent drivers from speeding. Where is the law of self-control applied to the speeding driver?

The way I see to fix the problem of high-speed accidents is to slow down the vehicles on the highways. It won't work by asking the driver to slow down, so it must be mechanically designed in the car engine. All the automobile makers have to do is install all vehicles with governors on their engines. Set the governors at fifty-five mph, and regardless how hard someone presses the pedal, the vehicle will only go fifty-five mph. The speeder who previously hadn't learned the powerful benefits of applying self-control when it comes to driving will. Not only will that driver benefit, but so will every other driver. There will be less stress, less gasoline consumption, less speeding tickets (if any), and a reduction in fatal accidents. The only thing we all would have to do is plan to leave earlier than usual—and that, too, is just a matter of applying a little self-control.

Self-control is the self-governing power, just like the governor on the engine of your car, that can help protect you from unhealthy desires, overindulgence, and making compulsive and irrational decisions. Having self-control keeps potential failures, unnecessary consequences, setbacks, and defeat from being a part of your journey.

Picture your life as a slide rule. At one end, you have obsession and/or overindulgence. On the other, you have neglect and/or abuse. Neither end of the slide rule is healthy, so both are out of balance. Self-control is your empowering ability to put on the brakes to bring your life into balance. Unfortunately no one has taught you how or when to put on the brakes or how to perform the balancing act. To govern and protect yourself, you need to establish certain standards. Standards are established through personal experiences, learning, studying and/or from examples set by other individuals.

To get the full benefit from the power within (self-control), you must set personal standards. Your standards may not be the same as someone else's, which is a characteristic of your individuality. But you must have your own standards. For example, I choose not to smoke cigarettes because smoking falls far short of the standards I have set for myself regarding my personal health and hygiene. By learning about the dangerous effects smoking has on my health, it makes sense and is compatible with my standard for my healthy lifestyle practices to be a non-smoker. If I didn't set a standard for my health, then my self-control would be powerless to me. Consequently, I could find myself joining the ranks of smokers.

Even in everyday life, self-control keeps us from harming ourselves in many ways. Think about how it is beneficial in these everyday situations:

▸ Applying self-control to drive the speed limit minimizes speeding tickets and helps keep you and others safe on the road—the standard for applying self-control is obeying the law.

▸ Applying self-control to budget your money is critical to be sure there will be enough to pay bills—the standard for applying self-control is money management and wise stewardship.

▸ Applying self-control to stay home and study instead of going out with friends to party decreases failures—the standard for applying self-control for studying instead of partying is maximizing academic scores.

Think about the consequences when standards and self-control are not applied for the people in the above examples:

▸ The driver has a much higher chance of being in an accident and/or getting a speeding ticket.

▸ The uncontrolled spender who lives for today could be broke tomorrow.

▸ The college student who didn't study will not score well on exams.

Self-control will become a key part of your defense arsenal for setting you free from the cycle of repeatedly making bad choices. It will free you from making the same decision that caused you to relapse and regain the pounds you successfully lost. Applying self-control protects you from related issues like having to deal with the guilt that generally is associated with failure and from feeling self-consciousness for regaining pounds.

> **Self-control is a built-in mechanism designed to protect you from failing to reach your goals.**

Self-control is a built-in mechanism designed to protect you from failing to reach your goals. It is a necessary virtue if you are going to be successful. If you make impulsive decisions, unhealthy choices, or don't take the time to stop and think things through before going forward with a decision, you will find the results of your decisions to be less than desirable had you applied self-control.

Using self-control is a powerful means of protecting you from yourself. It also promotes freedom, contrary to popular belief. Most people think of self-control as something that will restrict them from being able to do what they want to do or obtain what they would like to have. But the contrary is true. Self-control is very liberating and allows you to be in total control of yourself to make the best possible choices for the best possible results…for you.

When I am conducting seminars or speaking engagements on the topic of the power within, I generally ask my audience to give me their definition of "dietary freedom." The response is always similar. "Being able to eat what I want, whenever I want it, and as much as

I want." Then after hearing what they have said, I point out to them that what they are saying and experiencing is not freedom at all, but is actually a form of bondage and limitation. Eating without self-control in portion size, proper feeding time, or the food types leads to a myriad of health problems, weight gain, and emotional misery. That is not what I call being free. In fact, that makes you a slave to food. Self-control is the power to do what you ought to do, which in turns creates a sense of freedom—in this case, dietary freedom. By the way, can you remember the last time you did something that you knew you ought to have done for a particular situation and you didn't feel a sense of freedom?

> To protect yourself from falling into the temptation of overindulging, making impulsive decisions, or allowing your standards to be compromised, you have to apply self-control.

Setting Boundaries
Combat Twins for Protecting Your Personal Borders

The combat twin to self-control is setting boundaries. The act of setting boundaries is your defensive strategy for keeping outside influences or assailants from over-stepping the boundaries you have set for yourself. It says that you have drawn a line in the sand and no one (or nothing) is allowed to cross that line without consequence. It's another means of protecting yourself from negative influences by others who would compromise your standards whether they pertain to personal health and fitness, relationships, decisions for your career, money management, and others.

If a person did not learn how to set boundaries in the formative years, this person can eventually grow into adulthood with eating disorders such as compulsive eating, anorexia, bulimia, and overeating, all of which are often connected to a lack of boundaries.

Let me share a scenario with you about a grown woman with an eating disorder. When Susie was an eight- or nine-year-old girl, she kept a diary of the events of her day in her personal journal. She did this day in and day out. One day when Susie was not home her brother and a couple of his friends happened to go into her bedroom and found her diary. The boys opened the diary and started reading all of the events, feelings, and personal thoughts that Susie had recorded. The boys were laughing and having fun with the diary when Susie walked into the room. Needless to say, the boys freaked out. They knew they were dead. But instead of confronting her brother and his friends, Susie just sat on her bed and cried. She never did anything about it. Instead she let those hurt feelings stay deep inside.

Had Susie been taught how to set boundaries, she would have gotten in her brother's face, told him a thing or two, and snatched her book out of his hand. Had she done that, her actions would have been based on her personal standards she had set as to what she thought about herself. In essence, her reaction to her brother would have reinforced her sense of self-value and self-worth. She would have known that her brother was not allowed to violate those standards without consequence. Had boundaries been in place, her brother would have been more apprehensive about reading her diary in the future. But most importantly, Susie would have had developed a healthy sense of self love and self value instead of an eating disorder as a grown woman.

Think about this for a minute: *If you don't believe you have self-worth or value, what is there to protect?*

Boundaries and Forgiveness
"I love you, but…!"

I recall counseling a woman in her mid- to late forties. She was very attractive but her outward beauty was somewhat hidden because of her grossly overweight condition. I had her fill out a questionnaire so I could have some pertinent background information to help me. As we conversed she assured me that she was very much aware of what she needed to do to lose all that weight she had been carrying. But over time she had become extremely frustrated with the cycle of losing weight and regaining it. To add to her frustration, she hated the way she looked and how she felt about herself. She said she had tried everything. She had read up on all the latest exercise programs, diet plans, and she even took dietary supplements but her frustration was becoming overwhelming. "How could I make all these lifestyle changes, lose weight, and yet not be able to keep it off?" she asked.

After spending an hour or so with her I was able to determine what her real struggle was. I had noticed in her questionnaire that she mentioned as a pre-teen the fact that her mother was always on her case about her weight. No matter what she did or what she wore, her mother would ride her about her weight. As we continued in the consultation, I asked her about a statement she had made in her questionnaire about her mother. Her response was that her mother was still like that today. She told me that if her mother walked through the door right now she would ask "when I was planning to lose all that weight?"

I posed a direct question to my client. I asked her whether she had forgiven her mother yet. And if she hadn't, she needed to. She also needed to stop blaming her mother. The very moment I asked that question I saw these huge tears of pent-up pain start flowing down her cheeks. I knew that I had hit the real root of the problem. As she was crying, I began to explain to her that all the knowledge in the world wouldn't help her lose weight and keep it off until she addressed the root problem. In her case it was an emotionally rooted problem. As a preteen and even into adulthood she heard her mother's words over and over about losing weight, but what she was feeling was that she was not good enough to meet her mother's approval. And no matter how hard she tried to get her mother's approval, she couldn't. I am certain her mother loved her, but it was obviously conditional love not unconditional love. My client was held hostage to the pain of rejection from not being accepted by her mother regarding her weight all her life, ultimately leaving her with a broken spirit. My client would never meet her mother's standard of approval back then or now.

My recommendation was first to forgive her mother before she started to make any healthy lifestyle changes or she would just be spinning her wheels. Her comment was, "My mother would never understand why I would want to forgive her because she would deny that she was the problem I was struggling with."

I told her that her mother's response (or lack of) had nothing to do with forgiving her. Her mother was never going to change but my client needed to be free, if she was willing to forgive. I explained that it was her responsibility to heal and move on with her life. I told her by forgiving her mother she would begin the healing process from the emotional pain she was suppressing all these years. The healing process was necessary to establish a balance in her mind and preparation for establishing standards for herself regarding her weight and her health profile. From that point on, her potential for enjoying a healthy, fat-free life with emotional stability would be reached, but she needed to set boundaries. The boundaries would prevent anyone from crossing the line in the sand, including her mother.

After dealing with her emotions, she needed to establish healthy lifestyle standards for herself and apply self-control to protect herself from making those unhealthy decisions that in the past had caused her to relapse and regaining her weight. She has learned how to set boundaries for herself and for others.

To **Never Go Back** encompasses every area of your life. You must address the whole person. Self-control and learning to set boundaries are tasks you will need to develop and perfect. Your overall goal, however, is not to be perfect... but to make progress.

— Renewing Your Mind —

() Do you find yourself making choices that are impulsive and without much thought? Yes, or no? If yes, then exercising the power within—self-control—is imperative. Consider whether your decision(s) are based on what you "ought to do" rather than a quick, flippant response. Self-control is the power within to protect yourself from yourself. STOP and THINK before you respond or react to a situation, problem, or question. This will give you adequate time to allow your self-control to influence your decisions.

() People will invade your privacy, cross over the line, and violate you if you do not set standards for yourself. These standards are based on how you value yourself. Have you learned to set boundaries? Yes, or no? If no, then make it a point to re-focus on your self-worth and value. Like a valuable, precious jewel needs to be safeguarded, you do, too…but much more. When there is value, the standard is higher and holding any invader at the boundary line becomes easier. (Chapters One and Two would be good to review for re-enforcing your worth and value.) Remember: **you are worth it**!

() When your caretakers or other individuals inflict emotional or physical pain, it is hard to forgive them.

By not forgiving them you remain in bondage and are controlled by them. Over time, the pain turns into anger, and anger turns into bitterness. These negative feelings or thoughts influence your thinking and cause physical illness as well. Is there someone in your past you haven't forgiven, yet? Yes, or no? If yes, you must forgive them in your heart. Forgiving them is not to get a response from them but rather is a means to set yourself free! The healing process can not begin while there is bitterness and anger. Sometimes our pain and experience is so great and vivid that forgiveness seems to be an impossible option. If you find you cannot forgive them—for whatever reasons—you may want to think about seeking professional help to do so. Remember that you are loved. God loves you and people in your life love you. Remember to love yourself, too.

There is no use whatever trying to help people who do not help themselves. You cannot push anyone up a ladder unless he be willing to climb himself.

—Andrew Carnegie

Chapter

4

It's Time to Change

MY FAT TO FIT LIFETIME SUCCESS STORY HAS BEEN A NEVER-
ending adventure that began more than twenty-five years
ago. It wasn't built on a ninety day body makeover wonder contest
that typically starts off with fireworks and lots of drama, only to
fizz out faster than a glass of diluted soda. I wasn't writing a book
at the time nor had I intended to prove that I could lose those
extra pounds of flab I had gained so one day I could tell the world
of my success. My success has come from a change of mind, a
change of attitude, and a continual willingness to make whatever
changes are necessary for me to **Never Go Back** to being that 305
pound doughboy again. That's how important it is to me to stay
on top of my weight management game. That's why I have been

successful all these years. And that is how important it must be to you if you plan to **Never Go Back**!

So, how long should you plan to keep your weight off? What time line should you give yourself once you reach your ideal weight? I'll tell you in a nutshell: *Until you die!*

In this Attitude section, we have covered what I believe is the most pertinent area you will need to develop for keeping your weight off for life in this book—the gray matter between your ears. In the upcoming chapters, you will go beneath the surface to learn of the food triggers and emotional connections that are affecting your decision-making process. As you go beneath the surface, you will better understand the emotional connections that have caused you to either relapse after successfully losing weight, or how these connections may have prevented you from making progress and staying the course.

The information and challenges found in the Attitude section are intended to equip you with dynamic insights that you may not have known up to this point in your journey. They are absolutely necessary to implement if you want to be successful at keeping the weight off for the rest of your life. These mental/psychological tools cannot be touched or felt by human hands. They come from the hidden area of your mind—the seat of emotional consciousness—your soul. Developing the correct attitude for success is an intangible and invisible commodity you possess. This new attitude becomes an invaluable asset which will make itself apparent to those around you and to yourself as you develop it.

All the insights, strategies, and methodologies in the world can't help you until you are ready to change. Are you ready to make the changes necessary to conquer your weaknesses and past failures? I hope so. Just remember that you possess the power of the mind that will transform your present attitude towards yourself and your hopes for your future into a **Never Go Back** attitude. This will be yours with one condition only: Are you willing to change?

> This new attitude becomes an invaluable asset which will make itself apparent to those around you and to yourself as you develop it.

There is a famous saying that goes something like this: *If a person is not willing to change his mind, he won't be able to change anything.* So, in order to continue the journey to being healthier and more physically fit, you have to be willing to change.

Are *You* Willing to Change?

Because we humans are creatures of habit, change comes very hard. We have a tendency to gravitate to doing the same things over and over, burying ourselves in our own comfort zones.

As you think about the battle with your weight and/or your health, somewhere sometime you are going to need to make some changes in your lifestyle, if not for any other particular reason than for aging reasons alone…if you expect to live into those ripe old years with good health and quality of life. But you are going to need to make changes. It will be your decision whether they come by volunteering to change or by force. No, no one is going to put a gun to your head if you don't volunteer to change but if you procrastinate long enough it will be your health that forces you to make a change—if it isn't too late.

I have counseled many clients who told me they knew they "needed to change their eating habits…but!" Or, "I know I need to do something about exercising…but!" I don't know which person is worse off, the one who isn't aware of their health or weight problem or the one who says that they know they should change…but! The one with this type of mental attitude is, in part, a carryover of a crisis mentality that suggests if something isn't broken, then why fix it? Maintaining a healthy weight for life doesn't stem from a fix-it-up mentality, but rather from an intelligent, ongoing perspective of prevention.

My hope for you is that you will volunteer to change.

Change can be difficult for humans because we are creatures of habit. That means people tend to repeat the same things over and over—even if what they are doing is not good or healthy for them, or even if it prevents them from improving their quality of life. Unfortunately, most of us have grown into adulthood and have not been taught the importance of the willingness to make changes.

Developing the attitude to change or the willingness to change must be ingrained in our minds early in our lives. Regardless of what you are dealing with—whether it is maximizing your health, maintaining a healthy weight, and/or enjoying a good quality of life—unless you are willing to change it will be impossible to reach your full potential in any area of your life. So when should we begin? I say as early in life as possible. It needs to start in childhood. It needs to start with your children. The sooner it is taught, the more likely it will become a way of life for them, and not just a quick fix. Have you been that type of role model for your kids? Have you encouraged them that sometimes they will have to make changes if they want to be successful and get better grades? You can't expect them to have the best future possible if they haven't been taught the reality of the importance of being willing to change. They will get it from you if you are living your life that way.

The willingness to change is absolutely the key to accomplish your goals, your dreams, and to reach your destiny in life. So I ask again: Are you willing to change? Change for the good! Change for the good of those you love.

Motivation

You are in control of your health, weight, quality of your life, and your destiny—no one but you! In order to bring change—lasting change—in your life, you need motivation. Motivation is something everyone needs to make it to the end. By identifying your personal motivation for changing, it will be easier for you to make it happen.

Let me share a short story about a woman named Elaine. She was in her seventies and had never been married. She was a kind and charming woman and always had a positive attitude about most things. The major obstacle in her life was that she struggled with trying to stop smoking. She had smoked a pack of cigarettes every day for more than four decades. She tried to quit smoking many times, but she never experienced the long-term success she had hoped for. I think her problem was she aimed at the wrong target—her target goal should have been to "quit" not "try to quit" —there is a difference. (Perhaps she needed another reason to help her overcome that obstacle in her life?)

One evening at a seniors' dance in her hometown, Elaine met a gentleman named Melvin. He caught her eye and, in short, she fell crazy, head-over-heels in love with him. Melvin was crazy in love with her, too. The relationship grew, and at their age waiting was not an option. So they got married rather quickly.

A short time after the wedding and settling in their house, Elaine was sitting in her favorite chair out on their patio smoking a cigarette. Melvin went out to sit with her and they began chatting. "You know, Elaine, I didn't meet you until you were in your seventies," he said. "And I want to have as much time with you as I possibly can because I love you so much. And because I love you so much I have to ask you something. Would you give up those cigarettes for me? You know they're not good for you and I don't want to lose you."

Worried that Elaine would get all flustered and upset, Melvin continued, "I'm sure it must be very difficult to quit after all these years, but if you need help I want you to know that I am here for you."

Elaine was overwhelmed by those kind words. Elaine told Melvin, "For years I have wanted to quit smoking but couldn't find the reason to quit. Oh yes, I know about the health issues like lung cancer but for some reason I wasn't motivated enough to put them down and never pick them up again—until now!" Melvin was amazed and thrilled by what Elaine said.

Elaine quit smoking right then and there on the spot—cold turkey—and has not smoked another cigarette since!

What was the difference? Until she experienced the love Melvin had for her, she lacked self-worth and value. She lacked motivation. Even though she was aware of the health consequences of smoking, she still wasn't motivated enough. But since Melvin came into her life Elaine saw the value in herself and the value in their relationship. The rest was just a matter of staying focused on the purpose, and living a life of love and romance with a man who loved her.

—Author unknown

Check out the following motivational examples and see if any of these reasons can help motivate you to make the changes necessary in your life to accomplish your goals:

Reasons to Change

▸ Family relationships: The dearest of all people need your example. They need you to be at your best! You need to be at your best to be your best for them! Change for the good!

▸ Friend relationships: Be an inspiration and encouragement to them. Show your friends you appreciate them by example. Change for the good!

▸ Health: Have a better quality of life, weight loss, more energy, disease-free lifestyle. Change for the good!

▸ Personal: You need it. Feel good, look good, and feel good about yourself. Change for the good!

▸ Your future: An ounce of prevention/a pound of cure—a pound of prevention/nothing to cure. Change for the good!

Overcoming the Obstacles

Deep down in your psyche there is a battle that rages. In fact, it has been raging for most of your life. And though its existence is usually ignored, and for the most part it's subtle, do not be fooled. It is extremely potent. If you aren't aware of this inner competition going on you may never discover how to overcome the obstacles that present themselves at the moment of decision. These two opposing forces are vying for top position in your psyche. (Please note: I am not making reference to making moral or immoral decisions.)

One voice is the well-developed play caller, which, in most every case is the dominating voice you and I have learned to obey. This voice or play caller comes from years of receiving negative input into our subconscious mind. And since the subconscious mind makes no distinction between positive affirmation or negative input, the one which is most abundantly received can influence almost everything you encounter that requires a decision—especially when it comes to obstacles or challenges.

The other voice is the lesser of the two. It seems to need some personal training and deliberate attention. It is undeveloped. The reason this voice is the lesser of the two is because most of us have received more negativity from our caretakers (as well as from other people and influences) than we have had positive responses. Consequently, most people have to work at being positive and confident when they are overcoming obstacles and challenges and attaining their goals.

What goes into your subconscious mind will come out of your subconscious mind and influence your conscious mind. (Remember: *garbage in, garbage out.*) This phenomenon applies to both positive affirmations and negative input you have received, both of which have been stored within your subconscious.

Your subconscious mind is like a psyche library that has filed away all negative and positive input throughout your life. Those negatives and positive affirmations stored in that psyche library influence the words you speak, the thoughts you think, your self-worth, self-esteem, and your level of confidence to overcome any obstacle or challenge that presents itself before you.

Push the Right Button

I'm sure you are very familiar with vending machines. What a convenient way to get what you want at the push of a button. But the question we all must ask ourselves before we push a button is which button should we push? Will it be a bag of chips, crackers, candy bar, bottled water, etc.? In the exact same way as pushing that vending machine button, knowing which voice button to push will make all the difference in the world to you as you travel down the road that leads to reaching your fullest potential in body, soul, and spirit.

Let's examine both voices and see their unique differences so you will be better prepared to push the correct voice button.

NO Voice

The **no** voice is forever giving us the reasons (excuses) why we should not or cannot change. This voice interrupts other areas of our lives as well, and in most cases it plays a huge role in preventing us from achieving our goals, accomplishing things we are capable of accomplishing, and even worse, it prevents us from enjoying our lives to the fullest.

Remember that your parents or caregivers guided you through the formative years of your life. Throughout those wonderful, innocent years, it may have been likely for you to have experienced a constant barrage of negative directives or negative input. Things like: *I can't stand you. What's wrong with you? You kids drive me crazy! You're too fat! You're a lazy bum! Can't you think for yourself? Where is your brain? You'll never amount to anything!*

You may have a litany of negative input or experiences from your caretakers of your own, but whether you remember them or not, every one of them was stored in your memory bank. As your subconscious mind became filled with negative input, the **no** voice developed. Years later you may find it difficult to make decisions and stick with them, or maybe you are afraid to make decisions because the **no** voice (being the loud play caller that it is) is negatively influencing your decision-making process. For this reason you have backed down from challenging situations and haven't attempted to attain significant goals or started pursuing your lifelong dream. The control that the **no** voice has on you has prevented you from being all that you could be. It's time to stop pushing that button.

If you have tried to lose weight in the past and chose a particular weight loss diet to get you where you wanted to go, I guarantee you that you dealt with two thoughts: one, will this program work for me; and two, how long can I do this before I fail again? The **no** voice is the main influence that causes people not to tell others that they are planning on losing weight. By listening to the **no** voice they think they are safe from embarrassment should they relapse or not lose any weight. This kind of thinking sets the person up for failure right out of the box. This thinking is responsible for emotional failure, frustration, and discouragement.

Avoid NO People

It is easy to detect the individual who is controlled by the **no** voice. I refer to them as the **NO** (or negative) people. Their vocabulary consists of words such as: "No way;" "I can't;" "Not me;" "What if;" "I doubt it;" "Never happen;" "I don't think;" "I don't have the time;" "Maybe;" "I'm afraid to;" "I'm not able to;" "I'm not good enough;" or finally, "I don't believe." I'm sure you know one or two of these types and my suggestion is for you to stay as far away from these individuals as possible. They will only bring you down, dampen your aspirations, and get you out of focus. Can you imagine raising a child and using those kinds of words all the time? Could you expect anything positive to come from that child's life? Do you think those negative seeds sown into anyone's life would produce any positive fruit at all?

You have a choice! Do not push the **no** voice button!

YES Voice

Ah, the **yes** voice. This voice comes from your subconscious mind like its negative counterpart. But its inventory is not as vast. For the most part, many of our caretakers were not big on pouring positive affirmations into our minds when they were rearing us. Consequently, its vocabulary has been reduced to only a few positive words. This vocabulary needs expanding, and its volume needs to be cranked up a little, too.

The battle between these two opposites continues to rage. It is always going to be that way until you make a deliberate decision to push the **yes** button. That's when your life will begin to change for the good also. This voice always says, "**Yes**, go for it," no matter how challenging the situation is.

Understand that pushing that **yes** button may not be as easy as pushing the **no** button. That is true only because you have been programmed to accept the negative input you received for so many years. But by believing in yourself, you will develop a whole new attitude and ability to develop and listen to the **yes** voice when life's challenges come your way.

The **yes** voice is in a constant power struggle with the **no** voice. Once again, you can develop this voice by monitoring what you allow to enter into your subconscious mind. You did not have a choice as to the information you received from your caretakers as a child, but today you do have a choice. You can dictate what you want to store in your subconscious mind.

Avoid negative people the best you can. Refute all negative words and influences around you. Block the power of the **no** voice. Expose yourself to positive people. Receive all positive words and influences. Develop the **yes** voice.

When you push the **yes** button, your view of life's challenges becomes positive. The goals you set for yourself will become doable and more rewarding. You will have done more than just reach your goal; you will have learned how to overcome challenges and obstacles. You will learn to shut off the **no** voice, once and for all.

Once you give the **yes** voice precedence, it won't be long before you will hear yourself saying things like: "I can;" "I will;" "I will expect the best;" "I know;" "I will make time;" and "I do believe in myself."

— Renewing Your Mind —

() As you have read, children often grow up with a subconscious mind that has been filled with negative input. And as you come to making decisions by responding to the **no** voice or the **yes** voice, which voice you listen to will strongly determine the direction you take. Do you have special goals or lifelong dreams that you shy away from pursuing because you don't believe you can attain them? Yes, or no? If yes, then becoming aware of which voice you choose to listen to is the place to begin. Doubt and fear go hand in hand, and stem from uncertainty, unfamiliarity, and even past experiences. When they are dominant in your mind they prevent from you from believing in yourself and perhaps from attaining a goal you are easily capable of. When the **no** voice shows up loud and clear, ignore it and push through the doubt and fear barriers that have been holding you back. Soon you will begin to quench the fiery darts of the **no** voice through repetition of your positive affirmations.

() Is silencing the **no** voice and its negative influence a struggle? If yes, it may be you have developed low self-esteem. When you have been constantly bombarded with negativity, accepting a challenge can be very frightful. Let's face it, your subconscious library, filled with all that negative data, keeps reminding you that you *can't do* anything. ***Do not accept those thoughts!*** Your subconscious mind needs as much affirmation as it can hold. Use the following words as an exercise and speak them yourself regularly: "I can;" "I will;" "I will expect the best;" "I know;" "I will make time;" and "I do believe in myself."

() Have you failed at attaining a goal or overcoming a challenge because you did not want to make the changes necessary for success? If yes, perhaps you may want to consider the reasons to change above. Reviewing the reasons and their value for pursuing your objectives will fortify your attitude to stay the course. If you place enough value on your goal, it will be important to you and worth your time and effort. Be willing to change. There's no better time to change than now!

Section II: Emotions

Connecting With Feelings

Education is essential to change, for education creates both new wants and the ability to satisfy them.

—Henry S. Commager, American Writer

5

The Connection Between Feeling Normal and Being Healthy

Why is it that people can't, or don't want, to change? Remember *If it ain't broke, don't fix it?* This seems to reflect many people's mind-sets and their lifestyles because they don't really change until something major happens and their health is threatened. Suddenly this change is forced on them to protect their lives.

The Inner Battle

Once someone decides to change, it requires more than talk; it requires a radical shift in mind-set. We all know people who have talked about losing weight or getting back in shape for years, but when it came down to it, they were all talk and no action. Real change doesn't take place through reading about some fad diet or by using different words to describe what you are going to do about your weight. In fact, it's completely and totally impossible to experience lasting behavioral change *(doing things differently for longer than 21 days)* without understanding the underlying psychological dynamics you are battling inside.

This battle is between two extremely powerful forces that can be traced back to our deepest beliefs: those buried inside our hearts *(spirit)* and those buried inside our brains (soul).

> This battle is between two extremely powerful forces that can be traced back to our deepest beliefs: those buried inside our hearts (spirit) and those buried inside our brains (soul).

It is essential that you know the difference between these two psychological elements. The absolute most important part of moving forward is the point where you experience the liberating change that sets you free to **Never Go Back.** For those who choose not to, it becomes an insurmountable obstacle—one that guarantees that you will **never get better!**

You can read all the diet books you want, but until you understand how this internal process affects you personally, you will be helpless and powerless to change. Your failure rate will only grow, and you'll alternate between false hope and hopelessness.

When you break away from the cultural cycle of the "diet go-round" and take the time to understand these internal dynamics, your failure cycle will begin to slow down and eventually stop.

The cycle will begin to spin in a new, positive direction toward a better way of life!

This is not an overnight thing. It is a process that takes time because each person faces different challenges to overcome. There aren't three easy steps to experience a lifestyle that allows you to **Never Go Back**, but there are some essential principles and disciplines that can take you there. The first one is a radical change in your mind-set. Until you think differently about your health, your life will stay about the same. But when you begin to see yourself from a new perspective—BAM! Big things begin to happen for you!

I'm going to share some coaching insights and information to guide you past the mental barriers that have been blocking you from achieving lasting change. Real change begins on the inside, long before you can ever see it on the outside. Once you identify and begin to live out healthier beliefs about how you live your daily life, you will be halfway there. Look at the following powerful, underlying psychological forces to help you to understand and develop a radical shift in the way you look at food and managing your weight:

▶ One force is fueled by the very powerful emotional connection of *Feeling Normal*

▶ The other force is driven by the even more powerful dynamic of *Being Healthy*

Is "Normal" *Really* Normal?

Multiple factors can cause someone to feel "normal." But because everyone's definition of normal is different, it really means "normal to me." You don't think about it much, but you know almost every single element that creates your set of internal beliefs which affect every part of your life: home, work, relationships, finances, spirituality, and health.

Psychologists and behavioral counselors use more than one hundred variables to measure how you, as an individual, define *normal*. The box below lists just a sample of these. See how quickly you can spot how some of these factors have influenced your ability to deal with food, exercise, and a healthy lifestyle.

Factors We Use to Define *Normal*

Age, gender, culture, educational level, birth order, number of siblings, family background, personality, socioeconomic factors, religious beliefs, work ethic, marital history, community values, family of origin, work experiences, school experiences, failures, successes, accidents, illnesses, organizational abilities, friends, peers, professional colleagues, vacations, travel, holidays, teams, sports, concerts, entertainment events, geographic moves, difficult changes, painful losses, significant births, tragic deaths, traumatic events, wise mentors, patient coaches, caring teachers, loving pastors, gentle grandparents, reading books, mass media, television, music or film, childhood memories...and the list goes on and on.

Many factors lead to your idea of what is *normal* because it's based on a complex mental process. It's easy for you to grasp and sort through, because you grew up with those ideas and you live it. However, it is very hard for someone else to quickly know what is *normal* for you without some specific training and extensive education on the subject. If you aren't reading, thinking, or talking through issues with healthy individuals, then it's highly likely that you will maintain the same old *normal* outlook. This can actually be your greatest roadblock to ever experiencing lasting change.

Normal is our way of trying to describe things that feel comfortable or acceptable to us, and is one of the main factors that lead to shaping what we automatically come to expect from others—while we automatically accept these things in ourselves. Even if you wanted to change a part of your behavior that you knew was wrong and out of control, you would likely lose and go right back to the same old way of doing things without first changing your view of normal.

You probably are beginning to understand that *normal* isn't what you thought it was, which means that the opposite of normal really isn't *crazy* (as some people might describe it). It may feel *crazy* to do the exact opposite of what you grew up doing because you have always known that your way was comfortable and completely acceptable to you (even if you knew that it was annoying to the people around you). This is why some people throw out the words *health food nut,* as an insult to someone, and yet a healthy eater simply takes it as a high compliment. Others who are called *junk-food junkies* simply laugh it off as a joke and aren't bothered by the words at all. While both sides might be aggressively trying to communicate their point about the use of food, all the other person hears is noise because they know in their heart of hearts that they really are *normal*, and therefore all the other *normal* people in the world would, of course, agree with them.

All this confusion and miscommunication happens because of the very powerful connection between what is *normal* compared to what is genuinely considered *healthy.*

For example, research shows that 80% of American women don't like their body image, and many actually report hating their body image. Is it because they don't have clear skin tone, ten fingers, ten toes, two ears, one nose, and two eyes that can track light? (These factors are how hospitals score a newborn baby—by measuring the child's appearance and basic functioning of body parts using the Apgar scale.) Or, is it because they don't believe they measure up to the Hollywood standards of outward beauty and appearance—which is about much more than the right number of functioning body parts? The Hollywood scale is based on looking, acting, and behaving on the outside like a celebrity, instead of just acting like themselves and being at peace with who they are on the inside. If a woman embraces the false belief that a particular body image will guarantee acceptance and approval, she will never be happy on the inside because age and gravity will continually be working against her on the outside!

Now contrast that way of thinking with women in other parts of the world where these media influences aren't present. Guess what happens? You got it—just the opposite. Because these women aren't affected by outside influences, they don't worry about their body size at all. Why? Because the word *normal* to them is based on much more realistic factors, which reflect a much closer image to their own experiences, genetics, and culture.

Regardless of age, nothing really can change in a man's or woman's behavior or lifestyle until there is a change in thinking about what feels *normal* to the much bigger dynamic of personal beliefs that can lead us to a lifetime of really being *healthy.*

This very powerful (yet often invisible to us) dynamic serves as an autopilot in our heads and can trigger continual conflicts, habitual impulsiveness, compulsive behavior, or addictive relapses each time it comes up, regardless of our age. It is the source behind being completely out of control with our words or actions, even when we know better. It typically gets even worse over time if not addressed. It is what ignites the problems we have with others. This dynamic is the source of most marital fights, business failures, financial struggles, and endless battles with food.

Our invisible expectations may be quite visible to everyone else, yet silently they keep growing bigger inside of us because they're often fueled by our core beliefs and strongly held convictions about what is *normal* and therefore *right*—no matter how unreasonable or irrational these desires might actually be.

Feeling normal and being healthy are intertwined throughout multiple areas of our lives. They determine the base level of our self-esteem, self-discipline, and motivation. Once you can determine what a person will do in a particular set of circumstances, you can almost always predict what they will do again and again.

The Connection with Food

Hopefully, you have a better understanding of *normal* and *healthy*. Let's equate this to food. Sometimes, the most common problem for many people begins in their childhood. They begin to use food to *fix* other problems or pressures. It doesn't work because the focus is on using food as a form of problem solving instead of as nutrition to stay alive. Food can't solve complex problems for kids or adults. But if you don't understand the unhealthy connections, it sure can cause a lot of problems!

The changes necessary to help you **Never Go Back** are based on internal beliefs and core values. External changes like joining a new fitness club or buying a smaller swimsuit as some type of incentives doesn't work very long—if at all. That's why some people never seem to get better. All they have ever known is failure, frustration, and the hopelessness of **never getting better,** so they gradually give up on achieving their dreams.

They are not successful because they don't know what it's like to be freed from the psychological power of letting food control their lives, so they keep trying harder with the same repetitive process that only brings them more pain, difficulty, and failure—while their dreams of a healthier lifestyle gradually slip away and slowly begin to die.

There's a better alternative to dreaming about a balanced and healthy lifestyle: living it! That's what this book is about. This process has worked for countless others because it is built on a solid foundation regardless of a person's age, gender, culture, personality, resources, or educational level.

Good news! By reading this far, you've already taken some bold steps toward experiencing a permanent lifestyle change. Now you understand the internal dynamic that points you toward continual self-improvement instead of continual self-destruction. Now you're ready to move forward and learn how overeating can be triggered in a number of predictable ways—any of which can prevent you from achieving real change, or do the opposite and continually bring wellness to your mind, body, and spirit. It's time to take what you've learned and begin to move forward to identify the food triggers that have held you back. I'm ready if you are. Let's go!

> There's a better alternative to dreaming about a balanced and healthy lifestyle: living it!

— Renewing Your Mind —

() Are the goals you set for yourself such as losing weight or making healthy lifestyle changes based on (or influenced by) external factors such as TV commercials, peer pressure, or the Hollywood scale of outward appearances, or are they based upon what you feel is normal? If yes, then you may want to revisit the factors listed above that describe what influences an individual's viewpoint of *normal*. Your internal beliefs are strong, but they are sometimes undeveloped or are not implemented into your decision-making process, so the outcome of your decision to lose weight and keep it off may only be a repeat of failure and frustration.

() Getting a better understanding of what is *normal* and what is *healthy* when making food selections is critical to the your success of keeping the weight off for life. Can you see the difference between the two? Yes, or no? If no, remember that we all tend to resort to our upbringing and the way things were done. And that can feel comfortable or *normal* for us. But when you start applying your inner beliefs (even though it may feel totally opposite of the former *normal*), stay with it! You are not crazy! You are becoming more instinctive and in harmony with yourself, and you are no longer dominated by the external influences.

Getting my lifelong weight struggle under control has come from a process of treating myself as well as I treat others in every way.

—Oprah Winfrey

Chapter

6

The Beginning of a New You

LOSING WEIGHT RAPIDLY ISN'T VERY HARD TO DO ON A temporary basis, but keeping that weight off for a lifetime can't be done through a simple thirty-day makeover like many commercials and advertisements promise. It's impossible to go from fat to fit in a matter of days because fitness is the result of daily disciplines from healthier habits. Little things, done over an extended period of time, add up to a lot of change—the type of change that can last for a lifetime.

It's time to discover your hidden psychological motivations, which literally trigger your reaction towards food. Once you are aware of these inner drives, you can begin to make adjustments to build on your natural strengths, while you can avoid your personal weaknesses. It's time to develop the *new you* by unwrapping the *real you* through an evaluation process in the upcoming pages. The factors we discover will be the foundation to build on as you take positive steps to move from habitual self-destruction to regular self-improvement with a dynamic process that will give you the strength to **Never Go Back.**

Here's a foundational principle to grasp: You must understand the powerful differences between the *physical* and the *psychological* drives that affect your eating patterns. Once you see the difference, you can take action to successfully manage your own food triggers.

▶ **Hunger** is the actual physical need for food (nourishment) and can be measured medically through changes in your blood sugar or when you hear the powerful chemicals that make your tummy growl to be fed when it is empty.

▶ **Appetite** is quite different from hunger because it is based upon the psychological need to be satisfied on the inside.

One is about nutrition to energize our body's metabolism. The other is about trying to fill an inner emptiness that often has nothing to do with fueling your body. Understanding the real motivation behind our choices leads to developing healthy patterns that result in honoring our body with a balanced lifestyle of healthy nutrition, regular exercise, and healing rest. Learning how to identify your hidden food triggers speeds the process of knowing how to manage these powerful inner drives (applying self-control) instead of being controlled by your appetites or your impulsive desires for instant gratification.

Identify Your Food *Triggers*

The more you can honestly identify what your real motivations for eating are, the more power you will be able to access and redirect to have good health for the long term. This evaluation is designed to guide you through this very important process. Please take the time to get serious and think about how to respond as honestly as possible to enable you to identify the real issues that may fuel your hidden struggles with food.

Answer each question using a scale of 4 (to indicate the most important or most descriptive of your personality), all the way down to a 1 (to indicate it's not really important or it is the least descriptive of your personality). Remember, you need to rank each of the four choices to every question from most to least following this scale. You will be assigning a number to each option below the question, leaving none blank.

Scoring:

4 = highly important or highly descriptive of your personality or values

3 = important to you or somewhat descriptive of your personality or values

2 = neutral or depends on the situation and doesn't describe much of your personality

1 = non-important in relation to the other options listed; doesn't describe you at all

1. **How do you respond when someone at work regularly brings in sweets?**

   ____ You try to distract yourself to avoid the sweets by just focusing more on your work

   ____ You thank them and just eat a little bit so they don't get their feelings hurt

   ____ You eat it but feel angry inside because you think they are trying to wreck your diet

   ____ You don't feel tempted to eat the sweets yet are glad that others seem to enjoy them

2. **Which situations below might cause you to overeat?**

   ____ Trying to calm down or escape the stress and pressure of daily life

   ____ Celebrating a special occasion or holiday with friends or family members

   ____ Feeling lonely, empty, or upset inside over not performing up to your potential

   ____ I rarely overeat because of my personal beliefs about managing food in a healthy way

3. **What factors are most likely to cause you to just sit and watch TV?**

   ____ Trying to prevent feeling boredom by channel surfing just to see what's on

   ____ Wanting to see certain shows so you can intelligently discuss with others later

___ Interested in learning how the characters rapidly solve problems or stay in control

___ Experiencing different cultures or personalities to better understand their point of view

4. **Which approach is most common for you to take when you are involved in a confrontation?**

    ___ Directly expressing what you see happening around you to quickly calm things down

    ___ Trying to prevent the other people involved from ending up with hurt feelings

    ___ Actively avoiding the conflict to protect your own feelings from being hurt

    ___ Stepping back to quietly figure out what the root issues are that led to the conflict

5. **Which of these actions is most likely to give you the greatest energy boost?**

    ___ Doing something you really enjoy

    ___ Talking with someone you really like

    ___ Thinking about a positive experience from your past

    ___ Reflecting on your life purpose and personal mission statement

6. **Describe your typical experience with managing daily responsibilities:**

    ___ Feeling distracted, stressed or overwhelmed from having too much to do

____ Wanting to discuss and review your options with someone you trust

____ Detaching or pulling away from a situation to figure out what's best for you

____ Using a disciplined and structured process to stay on task with personal priorities

7. **How do you like to spend your free time?**

____ Planning or participating in activities which are fun and enjoyable to you

____ Connecting with friends or family you never get to spend enough time with

____ Studying or learning new things now to improve your life in the future

____ Quietly resting and recharging your energy without distractions

8. **When facing a problem, do you:**

____ Take immediate action to solve the problem

____ Ask others for their opinion or ideas

____ Think about which options feels right for you

____ Quietly pray about what to do next

9. **What factors would be most important to you if considering buying a pet?**

____ Pet ownership keeps you active because it involves some low impact exercise

____ Companionship from pet ownership means you would never feel lonely again

____ Caring for the needs of the pet actually makes you feel better inside

____ It gives you the opportunity to provide the pet a good home in a peaceful environment

10. **Which approach would you take if you had extra money in your budget?**

____ Race to your favorite store and spend it on whatever looks interesting to you

____ Thoughtfully select a gift to share with someone you care about

____ Buy something you have wanted for a long time and feel excited about owning it

____ Put the extra money into savings for a future "rainy day" when you might need it

11. **What describes your greatest desire in close relationships?**

____ To get to know other people involved in similar activities so you can do them together

____ To compassionately listen to the needs of others to better support or encourage them

____ To communicate effectively so others really understand how you feel inside

____ To teach or share your insights with others so they can find deeper meaning in life

12. **Indicate your typical response during extremely hectic or stressful times:**

    ___ Always feeling busy from trying to get it all done without burning out in the process

    ___ Trying not to bother others with your problems since they are having a hard time too

    ___ Feeling frustrated or confused with questions about why life seems so unfair

    ___ Resting in your personal belief that things always happen for a reason

13. **How would you describe your beliefs about exercise and personal fitness?**

    ___ An important habit that reduces daily stress and improves overall health

    ___ An important way to stay healthy which is easier to maintain when joined by others

    ___ A necessary but painful part of life best reflected in the phrase *no pain, no gain*

    ___ A rewarding personal discipline that develops physical wellness and strength

14. **How do you first react when hearing about a tragic situation in the news?**

    ___ Interested in hearing how the people involved reacted in case it ever happens to you

    ___ Feeling hurt or sad for the people involved and wondering who is going to help them

____ Worried or anxious about the possibility of the same
thing happening to you

____ Silently praying for the people involved to be safe
while hoping that things work out

15. **What do you think about most when planning holidays or vacation time?**

____ Finishing up home or work projects you never seem
to have time to complete

____ Having special times together with friends or family
while at home or on trips

____ Taking time off from the hectic pace of life to relax,
unwind, or have some fun

____ Spending quiet time journaling, reading, in medita-
tion or in mapping out future goals

16. **How do you usually respond when
forced to make a quick decision?**

____ Look at the situation and go with your gut instinct
about what you think will work best

____ Think about what the people you respect and trust the
most would advise you to do

____ Take the path of least resistance and agree in order to
avoid arguments or more conflict

____ Filter the decision through your core values and
priorities to reach the right conclusion

17. **How do you react when forced to make a major change at work or at home?**

___ Focus on what you can control and begin to anticipate and plan about what comes next

___ Ask others what they are planning to do as part of considering all of your options

___ Get mad at the people or circumstances that seem to be forcing this change on you

___ Accept the reality of the situation as just another part of life and try not to dwell on it

18. **What approach do you take when you begin to feel hungry inside?**

___ Eating anything as fast as possible in order to quickly get back to the activity at hand

___ Preparing enough for you and others, since it's likely that they are hungry too

___ Look for snack foods to make you feel better until you have time to prepare a meal

___ Stop what you are doing to prepare and eat a healthy meal and then get back to work

19. **How would you most likely define a healthy and successful lifestyle?**

___ Being self-disciplined, organized, and structured to successfully manage daily activities

___ Feeling connected to the people you care about and having regular times together

___ Feeling in control of your choices and having freedom
to decide what is best for you

___ Living in harmony with your personal beliefs in a
simple and peaceful way

**20. What are you the most passionate
about accomplishing in your life?**

___ Enjoying a long and healthy life full of meaningful
experiences and fun memories

___ Staying close to people by patiently providing love
and acceptance no matter what

___ Personal and professional success which brings the
respect and admiration of others

___ Living wisely and well to reflect God's love to others
in all that you say, think or do

Scoring your totals to determine your Food Triggers:

Now that you have indicated how important each element is to
you, it's time to go back and add up your total score by category
to get your final result. Here's how it works! Each question above
has four types of responses, which follow an exact format to
reveal four different quadrants that influence our health and can
trigger the appetite for food, which can be fueled by Behavioral,
Relational, Emotional, or Spiritual factors.

▶ The first response is always going to reflect your "B"
score for **Behavioral motivation**

▸ Your second response will always reflect your "R" score for **Relational motivation**

▸ Your third answer will show your "E" score for **Emotional motivation**

▸ Your final answer will reflect your "S" score for **Spiritual motivation**

Here's an example of how to add up your food trigger scores using the first question on the evaluation to show how to record and tabulate the numbers in each of the four quadrants.

How do you respond when someone at work regularly brings in sweets?

__3__ You try to distract yourself to avoid the sweets by just focusing more on your work

__4__ You thank them and just eat a little bit so they don't get their feelings hurt

__2__ You eat it but feel angry inside because you think they are trying to wreck your diet

__1__ You don't feel tempted to eat the sweets yet are glad that others seem to enjoy them

Using this example, the BRES scores for this question are:

B = 3
R = 4
E = 2
S = 1

This example revealed that the "R" quadrant was highest. This answer indicates that relationship factors were the underlying food trigger that motivated eating food to make someone else feel better instead of eating food to fuel the body. Now add up all of the numbers from each question to discover your total Food Trigger quadrant score.

Remember the responses will always follow the same BRES pattern on all twenty questions. Your score could range from as low as 20 up to a maximum of 80 in these four key areas to show your underlying motivations regarding the use of food, importance of exercise and rest as well as maintaining a healthy lifestyle inside and out.

Your personalized BRES scores go here:

B (Behavioral quadrant) =_____
R (Relational quadrant) =_____
E (Emotional quadrant) =_____
S (Spiritual quadrant)   =_____

Now that you have added up your total BRES scores, it's time to map out your numbers in each category on the food trigger grid below. This will help you to gain a visual understanding of which quadrant is most likely driving you toward making unhealthy choices with food.

Each quadrant can be understood in light of the following scores:

0-20 —not a major source of motivation to eat or food trigger

20-40 —mild source of motivation to eat or food trigger

40-60 —moderate source of motivation to eat and occasional food
trigger

60-80 —major source of motivation to eat and likely food trigger

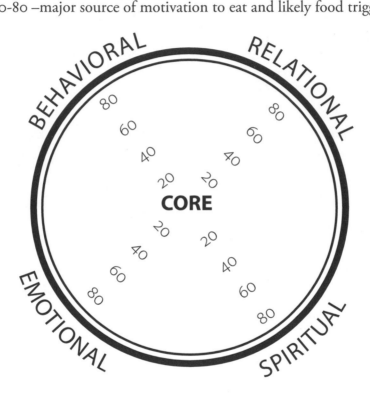

How does this graphic help me map out my food triggers?

Each of these four quadrants *(behavioral, relational, emotional, and spiritual)* represents a major factor that can fuel your psychological appetites and stimulate your internal food triggers. These underlying dynamics can lead to overeating in order to stabilize an internal mood or motivation that has nothing to do with physical hunger. Every calorie taken in during the food trigger process is eaten to satisfy a psychological craving, not an actual physical need for food.

Food triggers don't make you overeat, they just stir up the inner moods and motivations that can feel so uncomfortable that people frequently just eat something to calm down and feel better inside. Sadly, because many factors can impact your food triggers, it's possible to take in massive amounts of calories without feeling satisfied for more than a few minutes.

Now let's take a closer look at how these four food triggers could affect you and your ability to manage and control your own patterns of eating.

The top two quads are external and visible to everyone; the bottom two are more internal and harder to spot by others, especially if they don't know you. The left side is more about a personal view of situations, while the right side considers more about the views or opinions of others.

Back to the graphic—at first, it is difficult to understand the food trigger process with this basic diagram with four sections which don't even refer to eating or food usage. In order to get people to personalize this process to get serious about their quality of life, this food trigger process has been described in many ways. Men tend to see this as a target with the cross hairs at the core, while women have drawn it like a daisy with four rounded petals, but that's too soft of an image for some people to take tough action to change.

I once explained this process like a shamrock, but then I realized that being lucky was the worst way to communicate control over food because there is no luck involved in this at all! Luck is a temporary mind-set, while long-term success is achieved by doing the hard work of learning more about yourself to create a better legacy. Remember, if you don't really want to change to live a healthier lifestyle, you won't—no matter how "lucky" you think you are. Life doesn't reward luck. It rewards self-discipline and healthy choices. It always has…and it always will.

The best way to view this food trigger grid to really change and achieve better results is to simply see it as a steering wheel, because your life can only go where you steer it. It is similar to approaching a fork in the road in your car. You have to make a choice to steer the car one way or the other. Which will it be? If you over-correct or under-correct, you end up off balance and slide to the left or right as your life ends up out of alignment (at best) or crashed (at worst). The more you keep your life focused on a straight path and headed in the direction you want to go, the quicker you'll get to where you want to be—a place of balanced inner strength with strong inner convictions about using food as fuel to power your body instead of using food as the solution for fears, insecurities, or frustration.

No one can make you change *(at least not for very long)*. Even if a terrorist held a gun to your head and tried to force you to change, it would only be effective for as long as the bad guy had the power to control you…not one second longer.

Here's an example: A close friend of mine told me the story of how he and his wife were pleasantly surprised to win an exciting "vacation" at an exclusive south Florida resort that was frequented by celebrities from across the country. They were really excited when they arrived and saw the beautiful surroundings with all the amenities the resort offered. Unfortunately though, once they were officially registered they realized too late that this wasn't a fancy resort, it was an exclusive "fat farm" —a place where people were put through military-style workouts and forced starvation diets so they could lose abnormally large amounts of weight in short time periods. This couple struggled through the week—not because they wanted to but because they were locked in and the resort valet had stored their car off property to prevent them from escaping! When they checked out, they really were thinner, as well as sore and tired and more than anything else—hungry! Can you guess the first place they went? You got it—the first casual dining restaurant they could find with free bread sticks! After that, do you think they continued their strict regimen of harsh military-like exercises? Not a chance! **Forced change leads to frequent relapses.**

There's a well known phrase that says, "If the truth hurts, maybe it should." You might find that the "no pain, no gain" saying fits here…except that this kind of pain isn't about working up a sweat. It's about doing some honest soul-searching to discover the keys to a better way of life. A good example is the Biblical account found in the book of Acts, where blind Saul (later St. Paul) had "scales" drop off his eyes as he was healed, so his eyes were opened and he could see the entire reality around him for the first time which changed his life forever. The same thing will happen to you when you "see" the real you inside. Because when you see the real issues inside you, it's like you are really seeing what matters most in your life for the very first time. Remember, once you see truth, you can never un-see it. Just live it out and enjoy the journey of self-discovery.

The Core

In the exact middle of the four quadrants is the core. The core represents truth, and truth is the opposite of denial. This is where you should start when you begin looking at the evaluations.

If you are not completely honest while you are working on the evaluations, you will not reach your full potential. In fact, psychologists often recommend that a trusted friend, relative, coworker, pastor, or other confidante who knows you very well take part in the evaluations or scoring process because they really see and know that person. This person you trust is the person who can be completely honest and can often see things about you that you don't see. You want that kind of person because they care enough about you to take bold action to help you change something that seriously needs it. Everyone needs accountability from someone they can trust!

No matter what you find out, it's vital that you keep a positive attitude. The famous poet Ralph Waldo Emerson said, "Our strength grows out of our weakness." Right now, you may very well be like a student who can't figure out how to solve a math problem because they haven't been given the right formula to work with—with incomplete information the problem cannot be solved.

These evaluations can give you the honest awareness of your true motivations in dealing with food. They can't make you change inside, but they can guide you to change direction on the outside, leading you to a better place than you have been before—where you know what you need to do—and you have some healthy people around you to help you do the work to improve.

With this in mind, it's time to dig into more detail to understand each of the four quadrants that can trigger the cravings for food.

The Food Trigger Quadrants

Behavioral

▶ This trigger deals with known areas of human behavior and personal lifestyle. When you go to the mall, you can look around and immediately see things regarding a person's behavioral choices in terms of how they dress, talk, act, spend, and how they react to others.

▶ People who fall into this category tend to use food to have control over something in their lives, especially if they are feeling out of control in other parts of their life.

▸ Common Symptoms: Stress, burnout, always busy, never time to rest, insomnia or chronic sleep problems, fear of failure, financial fears, always worried about debt, job downsizing, unemployment or fears of unemployment, feeling overwhelmed in lifestyle, struggles with lack of organization or the desire to find instant relief, frequently at or near a meltdown in some area of life or they are racing to try and avoid the next crisis, tendency to be so busy with trying to manage their life that they never have time to sit down and enjoy any of it. Yo-yo diets are most common in this quadrant..

Relational

▸ This has to do with the basic way you connect with or deal with others. Are you outgoing and likeable? Do you smile at others or do you walk with your head down? Relational factors can trigger the habitual need to use food to find connection with something in their life, especially if they are feeling disconnected with the people they normally are close to. (It's common for individuals with high relationship food triggers to prefer to eat with a stranger than to sit and eat alone).

▸ People in this quad tend to see food as a connector *(like the correlation of how social eating can be very similar to social drinking)*. Frequent relational food triggers surround family gatherings, since every time friends and family get together food is the main connector. If a baby is born, the celebration must include loads of food, if an aged loved one dies, the funeral must include lots of food. They believe that every relationship is made better by food because calories create closeness.

▸ Common Symptoms: Misdirected love, loneliness, family of origin or generational factors, clingy or needy attachments, rescuing behavior, broken relationships, grief, loss, brokenness, rejection, hatred, bitter divorces, custody disputes, domestic violence, verbal or emotional abuse, fights with kids or extended family members, unresolved dysfunction or past family secrets in relational dynamics like abortion, adoptions, reactive disorders or attachment disorders from childhood. Tendency to struggle with feelings of approval from others which can lead to struggles with codependency.

Emotional

▸ This trigger deals with how you use food to avoid feeling any negative experiences or emotions that might change your mood or motivations.

▸ People who fall into this category use food to find comfort during periods of pain or discomfort in their lives, commonly referred to as *self-medication*.

▸ Common Symptoms: Unrealistic expectations, continually seeking excitement, poor impulse control, major struggles with self-discipline or self control, guilt, fear, depression, anxiety, isolation, phobias, panic disorder, grief, embarrassment, rage, moodiness, sadness, regrets, resentment, perfectionism, critical spirit, anger, trauma, PTSD *(Post Traumatic Stress Disorder)* and strong desire to appear emotionally 'in control' of any situation. Tendency to sit back and watch life through media images to avoid the fear of conflict in actually living life.

Spiritual

▸ Before we get into the specific definition on this quad, it's important to know that when we are dealing with spiritual dynamics, it isn't referring just to your religious beliefs. Spirituality affects every decision you make every single day of your life. Spirituality flows from your core beliefs and strongest values. Religion tends to be more tied to our cultural and childhood experiences. Every person from every culture has a specific system of personal beliefs that dramatically can impact their lives, but not everyone has taken time to really sit down to understand what this belief system means to them, and more importantly, what they can do about it to really evoke change.

▸ These are the people who, based on their core values, resolve to live a balanced life in harmony with their life's purpose and mission, and tend to use food as a nutritional source to monitor and balance their bodies as a part of creating calm contentment and inner peace.

▸ Common Symptoms: Driven toward self-less behavior, often can't take a compliment, afraid to indulge or enjoy simple pleasures, can go through periods of extreme self-analysis or loneliness, emptiness if not feeling on task, always seeking a deeper meaning, lack of purpose, struggles of maintaining a lifestyle consistent with stated belief system, mid-life transitions, always seeking to discover their true self-worth from a spiritual connection with God's message of acceptance and forgiveness, leading to deep feelings of belonging, connection, peace, joy, gentleness, kindness and self-discipline.

— Renewing Your Mind —

() Learning the difference between hunger and appetite is a good place to start when targeting those food triggers. Being honest with yourself is not always the easiest road to travel—all of us want to be seen as in control and normal. As you review and answer the questions above, is it difficult to go beneath the surface to find out what your weaknesses are? Yes, or no? If yes, review Chapters One and Two just to help you refocus on who you are, your value, and your purpose. As you reinforce your self-worth and value, you will find honesty is a road easier traveled than ever before. These tasks will become profitable tasks as you do some honest soul-searching to bring about change.

() Failure, guilt, and frustration seem to always fill someone's mind when they regain their weight, particularly after several attempts to keep it off in the past. One's moral score card is often the means in which success by weight management is measured—good for staying on the diet; bad for going off the diet. None of these have any thing to do with eating, or at least they shouldn't. This thinking stems from a dependency on a diet plan to save them instead of realizing the strength and power from within to win the battle. Did the results you get from the self-evaluation questions point out more weaknesses than you would have like to realize about yourself? Yes, or no? If yes, then you may very well have made a significant breakthrough for tapping into the strengths within. It's time to steer your life to where you want it to go.

"Only I can change my life.
No one can do it for me."

—Carol Burnett

Chapter

7

Moving Beyond Why

Okay. You have taken the evaluation to measure which of the four core motivations are fueling many of your choices about food. Now it's time to map out that data so it can be blended into your regular routines and become a daily habit to bring long-term results. This part of our journey is about guiding you to develop healthy lifestyle changes that will flow with your individual personality, not against it.

This personalization process is one of the positive results that comes from applying the **Never Go Back** principles instead of the old pattern of continually struggling with food by trying one frustrating fad diet after another. Every human being is created with internal strengths and weaknesses which require a personalized approach to experience lasting results. This may be a radical shift for some readers. This section is about guiding you to stop spending so much time and energy gathering volumes of information about your struggles with food and start taking positive action to change from the *inside* out.

It's time to move beyond learning more about it. It is time to just live it out and shift from information to application, from talking about it to doing something about it. I am talking about taking positive action to experience positive results because lasting change doesn't come from what you know; it comes from what you **do** about what you know. You already know enough about your struggles with food and weight control. Now it's time to move from the continual struggle to a surprising place. It is called *surrender*. Let me explain.

Many of us have grown up with unhealthy patterns and rituals associated with food. Since we are primarily driven by one of four basic drives, (some people can have a blend of two drives), it is essential to understand your food triggers in order to successfully manage your eating patterns. People tend to gradually lose the struggle with their internal motivations because this is a part of their basic personality. It's like fighting against yourself in an inner battle you can never win. This might sound like terrible news, but it's not. Here's why: you have the power to move from continual frustration fighting what you *can't* change, to investing your time and energy focused on the things you *can* change. You achieve better results when you stop fighting and begin to figure out the best way to flow with your strengths and avoid your weaknesses.

You Have to Give Up to Go Up...

Surrender is drastically different from giving up. Surrender is a reflection of the wisdom of an ancient prayer that has empowered millions of people to change over the last 500 years. It's called the "Serenity Prayer:" *God, grant me the serenity to accept the things I cannot change, courage to change the things I can, and wisdom to know the difference.*

Moving past the struggle to surrender what you can't change is not a sign of weakness; it is a sign of wisdom. Remember, many of the psychological issues that drive our food choices have nothing to do with calories, fat grams, or exercise. Carbohydrate and protein intake can't touch your soul. Food is only temporary, while your soul is eternal. Until you openly deal with the real you on the inside, you may stay stuck behind self-imposed fears and insecurities which prevent you from experiencing long term-success in achieving and maintaining a healthy lifestyle. When you understand the four internal motivations that drive your choices, you can more accurately take action in the right quadrant to prevent yourself from making the wrong choices. It's like putting out the fire of wrong desire in the right way: at the base of the flames.

> Moving past the struggle to surrender what you can't change is not a sign of weakness; it is a sign of wisdom.

Understanding your tendency toward eating from Behavioral, Relational, Emotional, or Spiritual motivations makes it much easier to deal with the real issues that may have set you up to fail over the course of your lifetime. When you tackle these inner forces which may be driving you toward unhealthy choices with food, you begin a process that brings lasting results because you are changing your habits and patterns from the *inside out* with a strategic focus on the real issues inside of you, not on some trendy celebrity fad diet.

When we understand the real motivations behind our actions, we can successfully develop healthy patterns to honor our bodies with food, exercise, and rest instead of being controlled by our appetites or desires. One of the most important factors to help you to maintain a healthy lifestyle is to know the difference between why you do things and *what* you can really do about it.

The Difference Is...

Those who always ask *why* deal with things pertaining to their past. They ask questions like: "Why do I do the things that I do?" or "Why can't I lose weight?"

Since you have completed the evaluation from Chapter Six, right now you might be ready to ask all sorts of *why* questions, too. But don't take too long dwelling on *why*. It's not constructive. It doesn't lead to achieving better health. Asking *why* doesn't bring about change. People who continuously say *why* often get bogged down in events from the past. They are so busy looking for excuses to explain their place in life that they never move forward to do something positive about it. Asking *why* focuses more on who caused the problem than who is responsible for doing something about it. This can often lead to more feelings of stress from additional hurt and resentment instead of building strength from the process of encouragement, empowerment, and strength. If you want to experience lasting change, then learn to ask *what* instead of *why*. Use this approach: "What do I do about it?" Asking *what* is more painful, but it's the path to a better way of life. Here's an example to illustrate the difference:

Phillip has always blamed his mother for his lifelong pattern of compulsive eating because she overfed him as a child. He has been stuck in the Emotional quadrant for years because of his inner anger, resentment, and bitterness over his painful childhood. His mother may never know the amount of inner anger he harbors toward her. It really doesn't matter because his bitterness isn't hurting her, but it's eating him alive. Instead of staying trapped in an unhealthy pattern of using food to cover the pain he feels inside while blaming his mother in the process, Philip could move from being stuck in the Emotional quad and move to take positive action in the Behavioral quad to focus on real change. He could stop focusing on the mistakes and regrets that took place decades earlier to simply focusing on the most pressing issue that would change his daily life. He could move from *why me* to *Now what?*

When Philip is finally and honestly able to face the reality that his mother isn't making his food choices anymore, he could move forward to take clear responsibility for his health without the distraction of the past getting in the way. He will be able to stop struggling with weight and food choices and instead spend his energy in a more positive way. He can decide what to eat or he can get some outside help in making those choices from many places: dieticians, nutritionists, cookbooks, sports physicians, trainers, nurses, or respected lifestyle and fitness web sites like www.Bodyredesigning.com.

There are countless resources available to choose from to find a better way of life when people really want to improve their quality of life, just as there are countless reasons they can come up with to be negative (and some of them may be very valid reasons). The bottom line is this: asking yourself *why* will never bring about the lasting change of moving forward. You must ask **What can I do about it?** If you are stuck in a pattern of unhealthy relationships and use food to cope with your pain and disappointment, you could be trying to medicate the pain of rejection or codependency with empty calories and carbs to avoid feeling hurt on the inside. Knowing *why* you make unhealthy choices will not give you freedom from a self-destructive pattern with food to hide from pain, but knowing **what** to do about it will guide you toward making some healthier choices, all of which eventually lead to a healthier quality of life.

There is no better illustration of this process than a two- or three-year-old child. Think about their favorite question. You guessed it: why! Often, even when the parent answers the question, it's followed by yet another *why* question. That's because their little minds are very curious and their world is expanding. Sometimes they aren't even old enough to comprehend the logic of asking *what to do about it,* so they just move on to the next *why* without really considering what the answer really was about anyway.

Meanwhile, once that same child reaches his teen years, he often moves from the *why* mentality to the *why not* mentality—smoke it…drink it…steal it…watch it…*why not?* They are at the exact opposite extreme from the toddler—they're only worried about having fun.

The process doesn't end there because when teens reach their adult years, guess what happens? They stop asking questions altogether and often blindly develop an "it is what it is" mentality. Someone whose family has a history of heart problem might say, "Everyone in my family has died of a heart attack, so it's going to happen to me, too," instead of taking aggressive action to make sure it doesn't happen. It's almost as though some adults reach a point of mental numbness, as they continually make the same mistakes again and again, just as American writer Henry David Thoreau once said that most "men lead lives of quiet desperation." This does not have to happen to you!

You don't have to stay stuck in the silence of a painful past. You are already proving to yourself and others that you are on a different and healthier path. You are reading about and learning this new process of life change. You have mapped out the driving force that fuels your impulses with food and you have discovered which quadrant you belong to. But that by itself isn't enough. You might find it highly entertaining to find out why you do what you do (or why someone in your family makes the choices that they make), but it won't bring about lasting change. Only when you ask *what* are you taking ownership of your life and moving forward in greater strength and purpose. You know which quad is most important to you, and when you know what to do to take positive action to change, you will. And you will move forward faster than you expected because you have identified which of the four quads works with your basic personality to achieve rapid results.

A story is told of a father trying to read the newspaper while he was being distracted and somewhat bothered by his seven-year-old daughter. To keep her busy for a while so he could read the paper, he took a full-page ad that featured a photo of a woman's face and tore it into many pieces. As he laid the pieces on the floor, he gave her a roll of Scotch tape and said to her, "Honey, when you put this person's face back together, I promise I'll stop reading the paper and we can play." He settled back and began to read again, thinking he'd just bought himself at least twenty minutes.

However three minutes later, she interrupted him again, holding up a perfectly reconstructed picture that, mere moments earlier, had been scattered pieces of newspaper on the floor. Stunned and somewhat puzzled, the father asked her, "How did you do that so quickly?" His daughter turned to him and said, "I turned the pieces over and there was a photo of the world. When I put the world together, the lady's face came together automatically."

The same is true for you and me! Lots of pieces in our lives may feel tattered and torn from past failures, but the good news is that you can put the pieces back together—and it won't be as difficult as you think to put your world back together, too!

Puzzle People

Taking stock of your life, or more specifically, your life experiences with food, is much like trying to assemble your own personal jigsaw puzzle. If you've ever tackled a complex jigsaw puzzle you know that it takes a great deal of time, energy, and effort to get the pieces together in the right sequence to achieve the right result. It's not easy, and a lot of people get frustrated in the process and give up.

When you initially open the box, you have hundreds—sometimes even thousands—of broken little pieces going in every conceivable direction. It is chaos, jumbled up in a box that never could become anything of value. So you just keep repeating the process of trying to sort through the pieces the best you can. Knowing your inner motivation gives you an advantage because it allows you to follow a particular strategy to move along faster with a new course of action. If you know how to patiently put together puzzles, you can learn how to manage the powerful Behavioral, Relational, Emotional, and Spiritual motivations. Here's how it works with puzzles, and the same process can work for you in mapping out a better quality of life:

First, you take the pieces and turn them right side up. Then you begin the process of connecting them together the way they belong. Once this time-consuming project is complete, you try to speed up the process by trying to put as many complex little "mini snapshots" together as possible. All the while, you are looking for "clues" you can spot from each piece. Does it have a flat side? Would it seem to fit on the top or the bottom, or somewhere in the middle? What colors or indicators would suggest that it fits in a particular section of the puzzle?

If you are patient, over a period of time you begin to see the outline of a much bigger image—an image larger than any one puzzle piece could ever possibly describe. As you begin to see the total picture take shape right in front of your eyes, it's not as confusing anymore; in fact, it becomes calming. And if you are fortunate enough to have the support and encouragement of a loving partner, family members, co-workers, or friends, you won't have to do all the work alone. Accountable relationships are where others come alongside of you to help you, and you return the favor by helping them. Both sides win because we can work together faster and accomplish more as a team than a lone ranger, who usually just ends up feeling lonely.

Once you get the outside border of the puzzle put together, you can more aggressively tackle the insides to fill in as many "blank spaces" as possible. Lasting change requires the same process. The more awareness you have of your inner drives, the better you can understand how they are released on the outside and what impact—positive or negative—you tend to make on others in your personal and/or professional life. Even with the insights you have gained so far in this process, you need to stay connected to your friends and family members, or with professionals such as trainers, nurses, doctors, nutritionists, teachers, or counselors, who function in the important role of providing honest feedback to keep you on track inside the boundaries of your own individual puzzle. By doing so, you can put the pieces together faster without being confused by placing things where they don't belong or, worse yet, spilling over your boundaries to confuse other people who may be starting to figure out their own puzzles.

As you continue improving in your ability to take these broken pieces and craft them into beautiful pictures, your self-confidence will increase. And each time you finish one puzzle in life, the next one becomes even easier to put together. Think about the similarities between people and puzzles. Many people do not view their lives as a beautiful picture; instead, they only see a box full of broken pieces with no hope of ever changing or becoming anything of value. Don't you believe it! You were created with a purpose and were given the strength of personality to make a positive difference in this world.

It's up to you to begin this journey of taking positive action to apply the insight you have developed to dealing directly with your inner drives in order to stabilize the areas that need the most attention. All allow you to achieve more stability, leading to less stress. If you are highly disciplined in managing your behavior, but cold and distant in relationships and use food to avoid feeling lost or lonely it's time to face that hard reality and make some positive changes. If you are motivated by spiritual values, but neglect dealing with the basic behaviors of daily life by paying your bills on time or taking time to exercise, you will miss out on the stability and success you could experience by building some behavioral structure into your life. You have seen what drives you. Now it's time to see what you can do about it, and take the steps necessary to self improve instead of avoiding reality and falling into a negative whirlpool of self-destruction.

The Process Leads to Progress

Some people view the process of learning what drives them on the inside as a quick fix, yet there is no quick way to develop a stronger sense of character and inner strength. It also shows how some people make a big fuss out of finally figuring out how to lose weight from eating less and exercising more, or the odds of getting sick decrease if you wash your hands before a meal. Some folks struggle for many years to move beyond the basics in facing their lives and putting the pieces together. They grow older before they actually grow up, so it takes longer.

Some folks figure it out faster because they develop systems, strategies, supports, and realistic solutions which are personalized to fit their inner drives and motivations. Be responsible to yourself by staying healthy and then be kind and help others as much as you can.

We all are on a journey and we all need to do what we can to help others take positive action to change, instead of being critical of them. They may take longer to move forward from the unhealthy choices in their past than you do. When they begin to figure it out, remember that it's better to encourage them. Once you begin to see the positive changes in yourself or others you can keep the momentum going by asking, **_what's next_** and coming along to add value to their journey from the newfound strengths you have developed on your own journey.

The **Never Go Back** process is effective because of its long-term commitment to building inner strength by using encouraging words, praise, and consistent positive reinforcement to protect personal growth. It is this process that leads to long-term strength and deep feelings of security inside. This is why it is essential to have a personal development program—one that stretches and expands the possibilities and potential of anyone who takes the time to sit down and map out their strengths and weaknesses in these areas. Once you identify the key areas for you to work through, it will be important to recognize those people from whom you might need to create some space or boundaries from if they continue to be cold, negative, harsh, or mean to you. Be respectful to others around you as you begin to figure out a better course of action and keep moving forward in spite of any harsh family members or coworkers who'd rather attack you than add greater value to your life.

Everyone knows that you should eat right and exercise. This isn't exciting news in the health and fitness world. However, if you take this basic information and begin to use it, your life will change dramatically! Your journey will go from an unhealthy spiral downward to a healthy spiral upward as the result of your healthier choices. Most people don't ever take the time to figure out their inner motivations and drives, and then begin to put the pieces together to experience a better quality of life, which is why they **never get better.** Figure out your puzzle. Begin to discover *what* you are going to do about it.

Never Go Back.

— Renewing Your Mind —

() Do you have a tendency to view life's questions from the *why* rather than the *what* perspective? If you answer *why*, then this is an opportunity for you to realize that you have the power to change things within you. You can reach your destiny when you start using positive words of affirmation, refuting any negative influences from others, and being tuned in with successful, positive people.

() Working through one's life's puzzle may be simple for some, and more difficult for others. Do you feel after reading the materials in Chapter Six and Seven that it may somewhat difficult for you? If yes, find that special person, or even like-minded people in a support group, to help you put it together. Many times people may feel timid or even embarrassed to invite others to assist them with more personal and sensitive issues. They tend to shy away from the support they need. But that kind of thinking comes from the **no** voice and you remember what to do with the **no** voice! *Focus on the purpose and not the task.* Assemble the puzzle by yourself, or with the help of others—just one more task in your journey to succeed!

Personality is only ripe when a man has made the truth his own.

—Soren Kierkegaard,
Danish Philosopher and Writer

Chapter

8

The Iceberg Personality Principle: What's Underneath the Surface?

D ID YOU KNOW THAT 90% OF AN ICEBERG IS UNDER THE water, leaving only a tiny amount exposed above the surface? Like an iceberg, a large portion of our personality is hidden from view. Most of who we really are is covered up and tightly protected from ever being seen by others. While it is normal to want to look good in front of others, it is not always healthy because there are many deeper issues in life that need consideration if we are to grow strong in our character development.

The Cold, Hard Truth

Hidden issues and character flaws under the surface can lead to habitual patterns of unhealthy lifestyle choices, causing many relationships to remain in a constant state of turmoil. There is a reason for every human behavior even if it seems to makes no sense at the time. Understanding the iceberg personality principle will give you a deeper awareness of why people do the things that they do. As you come to a better understanding of why things are really happening inside you (or the people closest to you) it will become easier to know what to do to break the pattern of hidden personality issues that lead to hurtful relationship problems.

> Hidden issues and character flaws under the surface can lead to habitual patterns of unhealthy lifestyle choices...

To find deeper meaning and experience healthier results in your personal life, begin by studying the two key factors in this area of personality development: Image and Identity.

Image Management (Skin-based)

The part of the iceberg that is above the surface of the water represents the *image* that we project to others. It's how we look, what we wear, how we talk, who we associate with, and how we live out our daily lives in words and actions. Everyone can see our image; however, to some who feel insecure or afraid of what others think, image becomes a mask to hide behind. This process is called *image management* because an insecure person will go to considerable lengths to avoid dealing with the deeper issues under the surface of their skin to get into their soul.

Some people spend considerable sums of money to change their skin with fad diets, painful surgeries, trendy clothes, expensive jewelry, fancy houses, or powerful cars to create the image that they are *cool* and *have it all together.* Others mask their insecurity by overcompensating in one area of their life, which throws all the other areas of life out of balance, such as over-work or overly religious activity at the expense of their health or relationships. Any behavior can become unhealthy if it is used to escape dealing with the real issues of the soul (below the surface).

The type of lasting change that brings the strength to **Never Go Back** cannot happen as long as there are hidden secrets, fears, doubts, confusions, insecurities, or selfishness buried deep inside. Taking action to move more of our real soul out into the open for others to see and know is like taking a big part of the iceberg out of the water and see it for what it really is.

Moving past the skin of what others see on the outside to openly sharing who we really are on the inside is a major step in experiencing the deep feelings of contentment—being at peace with who we were born to be. When you are real, you don't have to spend your time, energy, or money trying to act cool or pretending to be perfect. Then you have the freedom to invest those resources into really enjoying life, instead of just enduring it.

When someone is trying to pretend to be something that they are not, or is being an imposter to impress others, they are spending most of their energy protecting their image instead of growing and maturing into a healthier person. It takes a lot of energy to cover up who we really are. And, after a while, it stops working because eventually the lies are exposed. A clever or manipulative person who is living a life of deception may get away with it for a brief period, yet they hurt themselves since the truth will always be revealed for what it is. Better to live a life of integrity by being real than to live a life of secrets and lies that will eventually unravel to show selfishness, stubbornness, or arrogance. Remember, the person we most often lie to is ourselves. We can never experience radical and lasting change until we are willing to face the hard truth that may be buried underneath the surface in the darkest corners of our hearts and minds.

The image-conscious person is worried about looking good for a special occasion, not about feeling good for life. So they race through fad diet after fad diet, endure plastic surgeries, frequent the tanning salon, and spend megabucks on makeovers. Because these are just *skin-deep* solutions, you'll find these same frustrated folks hanging on year after year to the never-ending repetitive cycle of the next fad diet, major surgery, or tan salon visits—spending much of their money for little results.

You can either spend your time and effort on these superficial (*skin-based*) things, or you can invest into improving the real you (*soul-based*). The skin-based way of thinking better about our image is only temporary—eventually our skin sags and wrinkles.

It happens to everybody as a part of the aging process on the outside. Good news! When you begin to expand your thinking to actively develop your soul, it brings about a dynamic change all over. The overflow of healthy thinking on the inside surges into multiple areas of your life on the outside. You will have a new perspective about maintaining a balance in your life with healthier choices in the foods you eat and how well you take care of your body through exercise, hydration, and sleep.

Identity is the Key Issue *(Soul-based)*

When you catch a glimpse below the surface of another person's life, it can be shocking and disappointing. We've all had experiences where we became close to someone who turned out to be much less ethical or honest than we ever expected them to be. While it is disappointing to find out who is real and who is not, it can also be freeing. It can remind us that we all have character flaws and personality issues we need to change.

Sometimes seeing the flaws in others can be a way to hold up a mirror to see some important things about ourselves. Some people use these types of experiences to get honest about their own issues; they see the irresponsibility or self-absorbed behavior in others and use that information as a catalyst to make positive changes in themselves. Others spend their time comparing their areas of strength to the weaknesses and character flaws they spot in others as a way to self-justify or avoid the areas that they need to change in their own life. It is always easier to see the flaws and problems in others than it is to see them in ourselves, yet we usually need to see our areas of weakness more than they do!

> It is always easier to see the flaws and problems in others than it is to see them in ourselves…

In healthy relationships there is a give-and-take exchange of shared accountability and insights as to how to help one another improve and change.

Learning to look below the surface in ourselves to see the larger part of our personality is a huge step in our own character development and personal maturity. This process of studying our own identity can be difficult. We all have made mistakes and have huge flaws, which is why most people avoid ever dealing with it. As you begin to address the deeper issues of your soul, you will see that identity issues are a huge part of making peace with your past so that you can find enjoyment in the present—and plant the seeds for a brighter future…**Never Going Back.**

You need to begin to see your body as something to honor. Think of it as a place where you would be respectful, such as a house of worship, museum, or library. Regardless of your age or personal beliefs, you would instinctively know to show respect or reverence in those buildings. It's much more important to begin to see your body in much the same way and begin to treat it with great respect and reverence. Your life is a gift to be treasured. If your body is a valuable gift, then why would you ever fill it full of trash—internally or externally?

Integrity Is the Richest Benefit

When you follow the philosophy of *what you see is what you get,* you are getting real by allowing your *skin* on the surface of the iceberg to completely match the deepest part of your *soul* under the surface. Put into a one-to-one-to-one correlation, it looks like this:

Image = Identity = Integrity

The Bible says "a good name is to be more desired than great riches," because of the importance of having personal integrity over every other characteristic. Getting real with who you are in the deepest parts allows you to have the courage to move beyond the insecurities and fears that have been holding you back. As you become more focused on living consistently with balance between your image *(skin)* and your true identity *(soul),* you will dramatically increase the personal integrity and strength of character to **Never Go Back!**

The most important part of life is trust, because trust is everything. With trust, everything is possible; without it, nothing is possible. Each time you take bold action to face and deal with the issues under the surface, you will experience a greater contentment on the inside and a greater sense of confidence with others on the outside. Every time you decide to make the choice to move forward in dealing with the deeper issues of life, you will mature and grow stronger to face your fears and insecurities. This process of facing issues instead of avoiding them will cause you to build integrity in all other areas of life, which will either feel terrifying or freeing. It all depends upon how well you understand the spiritual applications of sorting through emotions to discover the character issues and life applications underneath.

No matter how frustrated or defeated you have felt about your food choices or your inability to manage weight, remember this important insight. If you stop spending your energy trying to change the people in your life who don't want to change, you can discover a hidden source of power for personal change in your own life. You can allow difficult people or painful experiences to crush you, or you can allow those same people and experiences to radically challenge and develop your personal growth and ability to change. Just remember to move from *why* to *what you are going to do about it.*

▶ It's not about how mean they are; it's about how maturely you are going to handle it.

▶ It's not about their harsh criticisms; it's about your ability to make healthy choices.

▶ It's not about how much they argue; it's about how you will take positive action.

There are no shortcuts to this type of character development and personal maturity; however, there are several ways to move faster through the process.

The first is spiritual, based on finding a deeper level of **insight** into the agenda and real motivations of the heart. Put bluntly, it is prime time to deal with the underlying character issues that may have needed your attention for a long time. King David ruled over ancient Israel thousands of years ago. Listen to the honesty that flows from his soul in this verse from Psalm 139: "Search me O God and know my heart. Test me and show my anxious thoughts. See if there is any wicked way in me and lead me in the way everlasting." David is remembered as one of the greatest leaders of all time because of his remarkable honesty and integrity. His prayer revealed the insight to face his frustrations and enabled him to move beyond his fears and find a deeper faith in God. Like David, you must face your innermost feelings and issues.

The second way to experience growth and change is through the cognitive process of gathering *information* and seeking the truth about our issues by building new strategies that can bring positive change. This data could come from books, tapes, CDs, seminars, DVDs, training sessions, radio broadcasts, blogs, newsletters, magazines, workbooks, podcasts, films, or television programs focused on growth and accountability. There is a wealth of information available through public libraries, hospitals, clinics, churches, clergy, counselors, and the internet (to some degree). (Note: Not everything you read on the internet is accurate, so remember to always check the source of your research to prevent you from drawing any wrong conclusions.) No matter where you find it, get started now on seeking out the sources of positive information that will lead you toward taking action to change.

The third approach is built on *intimacy*, but not the kind you might think of when you first hear that word. I'm talking about the intimacy of being very close to people who care about you and you care about them. Human beings were made to be in close personal relationships so that we can help one another change and grow. Lonely people miss out on the benefit and value of knowing they are growing closer to others. Given a chance to help others spot and work through their character issues, they could someday receive that help in return. This is where the remarkable value of small groups is most useful in experiencing a life of lasting change. Being around others who will remain compassionate but still ask the hard questions about why you aren't changing in your use of food or lack of exercise will challenge you to stay on track in the important work of growing stronger in your soul. Then you can overcome the old food temptations that used to be stirred up by weaknesses and impulsivity.

To experience a better life you have to move from the surface issues in life and go deep into the issues of the soul. The more you take positive action to focus on the deeper areas of the iceberg, the more that will be revealed to you. When you are serious about change, it will happen. But keep in mind the old saying, "There is no testimony without a test." You will be challenged if you want to get real and deal with the deeper issues inside that may have led to a pattern of avoidance, denial, minimizing, justifying, or lying about not having problems. You could fail by trying to face these fears alone. Or, you could reach out to others to allow them to help you on the journey. You will have a better quality of life because you made the choice to face whatever is in your path with God's help and the assistance of healthy people. These people are usually not too far away if we allow them to come along with us and make a difference in our lives.

Begin with where you are by assessing your life today. As you move forward, take the insights you discovered in reading these pages and apply them to other areas of your life, too. I challenge you to make every effort to get real in building a life of personal insight from a deeper level of personal integrity. As you learn to master the process of lifelong change, it will be significantly easier to find the energy to do the right thing in parenting, partnering, and being the leader that you were designed to become at work or home. No longer wearing a mask and trying to cover up the deeper issues in life, you will have learned to become completely free to move beyond tip of the iceberg to live out your true identity in the peace and contentment that only those who are real ever get to experience. That's a life that **Never Goes Back,** and that's the kind of lifestyle where you are so busy enjoying the journey that there isn't much time for any thing else.

— Renewing Your Mind —

() Sometimes the truth about ourselves can be embarrassing and awkward if revealed to others. Fears, insecurities, etc. can cause us to put on a front or live a skin-based life—trying to be perfect instead of being real. Do you have a tendency to cover up the outside so no one can tell who the real person is on the inside? Yes, or no? If yes, then it is the perfect time to go under the surface and confront those areas you are trying to hide from others so you can reveal the real person. Revisit the iceberg principle and work on being honest with yourself. We all should take a long look into the mirror, so we can see what needs to be improved on. Every one of us has character flaws and shortcomings. No one person has it all together—all the time! Your goal is to go beneath the surface so you can identify your individuality and uniqueness to improve on yourself, not spend your life trying to be perfect.

() When we are trying to hide those areas of our lives that need to be developed or changed, we may find ourselves looking at other people and their flaws. It seems easy to see the flaws in others while at the same time nearly impossible to see our own. When you see flaws in others, do you make it an opportunity to do some soul-searching? Yes, or no? If no, then remember that to develop more character and integrity and honesty with ourselves we need to go beneath the surface. Realize that integrity and honesty are wonderful attributes for others to see in us. Your development and growth will not only make your life richer and with more purpose, but it could be a light for someone who is still in darkness. A superficial skin-based person is not revealing the true person to others. This person consequently suffers from the lack of deep contentment and happiness that is theirs to own. As you search your spiritual perspective and you look at your own flaws, you are sure to have a better character-building experience. Look at your own flaws honestly...not those of others.

Section III: Diet

Instinctive Eating

*One should eat to live,
not live to eat.*

—Cicero

Chapter

9

Your Weight And Your Health

ONE IN THREE AMERICAN ADULTS (OR FIFTY-EIGHT MILLION) from age twenty through age seventy-four are overweight. Obesity is associated with nearly 822 deaths per day in America and costs the country more than $240 billion in obesity-related illnesses. "Only smoking exceeds obesity in its contribution to total mortality rates in the United States. The nation can no longer afford to ignore obesity as a major medical problem," says Dr. William Dietz, director of Nutrition and Physical Activity for Disease Control and Prevention. Being overweight and physically inactive account for more than 300,000 premature deaths each year in the United States, second only to tobacco-related deaths. "Obesity and overweight are linked to the nation's number one killer—heart disease—as well as diabetes and other chronic conditions," says Jeffrey P. Koplan, director of the Centers for Disease Control (CDC). Besides increasing the risks for heart disease and diabetes, obesity increases the risk of developing high blood pressure, stroke, and gallbladder disease.

Our children have become victims as well. The American lifestyle of inactivity has played a devastating role on the children of our country. Now, eleven percent of our children are overweight or obese. Research has shown that sixty percent of overweight five- to ten-year-old children have at least one risk factor for heart disease, hyperlipidemia, and elevated blood pressure or insulin levels.

I can't tell you how many times I have counseled men in their late thirties and mid-forties who are recovering from recent heart attacks who have told me they wished they would have listened to all the advice they received—including losing excess weight—prior to their heart attacks. Yet the October 13, 1999, issue of *JAMA* showed that two-thirds of adults attempting to lose weight or keep from gaining it would rather take the weight loss lotions, potions, and pills than to follow sound, sensible guidelines that have the best chance of producing long-lasting results. Without definite lifestyle changes, all the fad diets will only provide temporary results at best. The weight will keep coming back.

Studies show that an obese person generally dies prematurely, deals with heart disease for upwards of twelve to fifteen years, and has more trips to the hospital—and therefore more medical bills. Statistics indicate that an obese person can actually expect to add twenty quality years to his or her life simply by losing the excess weight.

Who is at Risk?

Perhaps you wonder if the extra fat you may be carrying is affecting you. Let's look at some ways to determine that.

The standards for measuring obesity or being overweight have changed in the last years. One way to determine obesity today is to use the body-mass index (BMI), which is a method of comparing height to weight. See chart on next page.

According to this chart, a person who is five feet, eight inches tall and weighs 140 pounds would have a BMI of 21. A BMI of 19 to 24.9 is considered to be within the normal range, while a BMI reading of 25 to 29.9 is considered to be overweight. Any reading over 30 is considered obese. Researchers who use this standard estimate that more than one-half of the adult America population is either obese or overweight! This approach does not factor in the individual's muscle development or lean muscle mass.

In my opinion, using just height and weight is simplifying it too much. Too many times I have seen men or women virtually panic over what the scale reads when in fact, the scale is the worst and most inaccurate method of monitoring weight. We could place potatoes or bricks or a person on a scale and read 150 on the dial. The scale tells us nothing about the quality or condition of that weight. In other words, a person could look great at 150 pounds, or a person could look terrible at that weight. It is all determined by the composition of the body.

My preference for determining whether a person is overweight or obese is using a body-mass index that measures body fat

Body Mass Index Chart

Weight (lbs)	4'10"	4'11"	5'0"	5'1"	5'2"	5'3"	5'4"	5'5"	5'6"	5'7"	5'8"	5'9"	5'10"	5'11"	6'0"	6'1"	6'2"	6'3"	6'4"
100	21	20	20	19	18	18	17	17	16	16	15	15	14	14	14	13	13	13	12
105	22	21	21	20	19	19	18	18	17	16	16	16	15	15	14	14	14	13	13
110	23	22	22	21	20	20	19	18	18	17	17	16	16	15	15	15	14	14	13
115	24	23	23	22	21	20	20	19	19	18	18	17	17	16	16	15	15	14	14
120	25	24	23	23	22	21	21	20	19	19	18	18	17	17	16	16	15	15	15
125	26	25	24	24	23	22	22	21	20	20	19	18	18	17	17	17	16	15	15
130	27	26	25	25	24	23	22	22	21	20	20	19	19	18	18	17	17	16	16
135	28	27	26	26	25	24	23	23	22	21	21	20	19	19	18	18	17	17	16
140	29	28	27	27	26	25	24	23	23	22	21	21	20	20	19	19	18	18	17
145	30	29	28	27	27	26	25	24	23	23	22	21	21	20	20	19	19	18	18
150	31	30	29	28	27	27	26	25	24	24	23	22	22	21	20	20	19	19	18
155	32	31	30	29	28	28	27	26	25	24	24	23	22	22	21	20	20	19	19
160	34	32	31	30	29	28	28	27	26	25	24	24	23	22	22	21	21	20	20
165	35	33	32	31	30	29	28	28	27	26	25	24	24	23	22	22	21	21	20
170	36	34	33	32	31	30	29	28	27	27	26	25	24	24	23	22	22	21	21
175	37	35	34	33	32	31	30	29	28	27	27	26	25	24	24	23	23	22	21
180	38	36	35	34	33	32	31	30	29	28	27	27	26	25	24	24	23	23	22
185	39	37	36	35	34	33	32	31	30	29	28	27	27	26	25	24	24	23	23
190	40	38	37	36	35	34	33	32	31	30	29	28	27	27	26	25	24	24	23
195	41	39	38	37	36	35	34	33	32	31	30	29	28	27	27	26	25	25	24

percentage against the lean body or muscle weight. This method of determining body composition says much more than just weight does because it relates directly to health. (Most YMCAs, health clubs, and health fairs offer body fat testing.)

A female is considered clinically obese when her body fat is thirty percent or greater. A male is considered clinically obese when his body fat surpasses twenty-five percent. The good news is that people can change their body composition through fitness programs, sports, and physical activities that stimulate muscle growth. The amount they weigh can become composed of less fat and more muscle. I believe the BMI measuring gives a more accurate representation of health.

The Obesity-Disease Connection

"Malignant obesity" is a term now used to define persons sixty percent above desirable weight; this corresponds to an absolute excess of 100 pounds. With this degree of obesity, there is at least a doubling of all causes of morbidity and mortality. Obese people who are diabetic or who have hypertension, heart disease, or any other cardiovascular disease risk factor **must** reduce their weight. It is truly a matter of life or death.

Hypertension, or high blood pressure, is commonly associated with obesity. Overweight men and women from the age twenty to their mid-forties are six times more likely to have hypertension than their same-aged peers of normal weight. Weight gain in young adults sets the stage for hypertension in later years.

Menopausal women whose excess fat has been localized in the upper torso (upper back, arms, and stomach) have an increased risk of developing breast cancer. Overweight women also higher rates of cancer of the uterus and ovaries. Overweight men have a definite higher mortality rate for colorectal and prostate cancers.

Being overweight places unnecessary trauma on the weight-bearing joints such as the knees. In middle-aged women, excess body weight is a major predictor of osteoarthritis of the knees. Every time overweight people reduce their body weight, they are increasing the longevity of their joints while improving their mobility to perform everyday tasks.

The Obesity-Psychological Disorders Connection

Because of their excess weight and size, many obese individuals suffer from lower back and joint pain and inflammation. They may also have difficulty breathing. Overweight people may struggle with issues of inadequacy or lowered self-worth related to their performance of normal day-to-day tasks at work, play, or social interaction.

> Overweight people may struggle with issues of inadequacy or lowered self-worth related to their performance…

Additionally, people struggling with obesity may have felt discriminated against at one time or another, possibly in a work or academic setting.

These psychological issues that are associated with poor body image are often a consequence of obesity.

The Obesity-Diabetes Connection

Nearly eighty percent of patients with non-insulin-dependent diabetes mellitus are obese. Many people with this type diabetes struggle with weight gain due to the lack of regular exercise. Since the body is not burning or metabolizing calories adequately, it stores them in the form of fat.

Excess body fat interferes with normal blood glucose levels. Because the body no longer handles insulin normally, the blood sugar or glucose builds up in the blood, and blood glucose levels increase. This generally is due to overeating or eating too much at one time. Regular exercise and weight loss will help to normalize the blood sugar levels.

High-Glycemic Foods and Weight

Over the years I have asked hundreds of clients and students to fill out a three-day dietary analysis of the foods and beverages they consume. From these, I noticed a common denominator: Most of them selected high-glycemic foods for over eighty percent of their diets!

High-glycemic foods are simple sugars or carbohydrates. They consist of single sugar molecules that convert to energy very quickly. When ingested, they provide immediate energy, which is great when a person is in need of raising glucose levels or requires an immediate lift for performing a task. But when too many high-glycemic foods are consumed, they can play havoc on our metabolisms by slowing down the body's ability to burn calories and causing hypoglycemia, or low blood sugar.

Many people have been led to believe that a diet high in carbohydrates is healthy. But from all of my findings, both personally and professionally, I believe that most people are carrying too much body fat and are unhealthy because they are eating too many carbohydrates.

Typically, a glycemic index food chart lists the conversion rate of a food to energy, or how much the insulin level increases when that food is ingested. After food is ingested, the pancreas produces insulin. Insulin then does its job and transports truckloads of sugar over to the furnace (or power plant) in the cell to be burned. These power plants, called mitochondria, convert the sugar into usable energy. When too many simple sugars are ingested, the power plant becomes full. Then the overflow is stored in the liver and fat cells. This is not something you want if you are trying to lose weight! Too many simple sugars eaten day after day can also contribute to diabetes and other health problems. (See the explanation above concerning those problems.)

Insulin's normal function is to escort glucose to your cells for energy conversion. A continual over-insulin response caused by the over-consumption of simple sugars (high-glycemic food) encourages fat storage. It causes low blood sugar, slows your metabolism, makes you tired and hungry, weakens your immune system, and interferes with protein synthesis (your body's ability to build muscle or lean weight).

Foods on the glycemic food chart are rated by number from 0 to 100, with 100 representing how high the insulin rises when straight glucose (sugar) is ingested. The foods with higher numbers are high-glycemic or quick-energy foods such as candy bars, breads, juice, white bread, white rice, corn, and sweeteners such as corn syrup, to name a few.

If you are like most Americans today and get the majority of your calories from high-glycemic foods, then you are flirting with potential health and weight problems. To better control sugar cravings, stabilize blood sugar levels, promote weight loss, and have more energy throughout each day, eat low-glycemic foods as your staple.

(Use the lists in this chapter for reference when selecting low-glycemic foods and avoiding high-glycemic foods.)

Glycemic Index for Selected Carbohydrates

The higher the glycemic index, the more significant effect a particular food will have on your blood sugar.

- Glucose 100
- Baked Potatoes 95
- White Bread 95
- Mashed Potatoes 90
- Honey 90
- Carrots 85
- Corn Flakes, popcorn 85
- Refined cereal (with sugar) 70
- Chocolate bar, candy bar 70
- Cookies 70
- Boiled potatoes 70
- White rice 70
- Corn 70
- Half bread (half white, half whole grain) 65
- Beets 65
- Banana 60
- Jam 55
- White Pasta 55
- Whole grain bread 50
- Complete cereal (no sugar) 50
- Oat Flakes 40
- Fresh fruit juice (no sugar) 40

- ▶ **Rye bread** 40
- ▶ **Dairy** 35
- ▶ **Dry beans** 30
- ▶ **Lentils** 30
- ▶ **Garbanzo beans** 30
- ▶ **Fresh fruit** 30
- ▶ **Fruit marmalade (no sugar)** 25
- ▶ **Fructose** 20
- ▶ **Dark chocolate (more than 60% cocoa)** 22
- ▶ **Soy** 15
- ▶ **Green veggies, tomatoes, lemon, mushrooms less than** 10

High-Glycemic Foods

▸ Foods containing sugar, honey, molasses, and corn syrup

▸ Fruits such as bananas, watermelon, pineapple, and raisins

▸ Vegetables such as potatoes, corn, carrots, beets, turnips, and parsnips

▸ Breads such as all-white breads, all-white flour products, and corn breads

▸ Grains including rice, rice products, millet, corn, and corn products

▸ Pasta, especially thick, large pasta shapes

▸ Cereals, including all cereals except those on the low-glycemic list below

▸ Snacks, especially potato chips, corn chips, popcorn, rice, cakes, and pretzels

▸ Alcoholic beverages

Low-Glycemic Foods

▸ Foods sweetened with saccharin, aspartame, or fructose
▸ All meats
▸ All dairy products (no sugars)
▸ Fruits, except the high-glycemic fruits listed
▸ Vegetables, except the high-glycemic vegetables listed
▸ Breads such as whole rye, pumpernickel, and whole-wheat pita
▸ Grains, including barley, bulgur, and kasha
▸ Pasta, such as thin strands, whole-wheat pasta, and lean threads
▸ Cereals like Special K, All Bran, Fiber One, and regular oatmeal
▸ Snacks, including nuts, olives, cheese, and pita chips
▸ Red wine

Low-Glycemic Food Choices

It was interesting to observe the connection between the food choices my students recorded and the symptoms about which they complained: light-headed, dizziness, brain fog, overweight to obesity, sugar cravings, and sometimes depression and irritability.

John attended my Fitness and Fellowship class. During one of our classes, he told all of us that after he had eaten breakfast, he found it nearly impossible to keep his eyes open. By the time he drove to work he felt terrible. I asked him what he had been eating for breakfast. "Sometimes cereal and milk, or sometimes toast and coffee. But I always have a big glass of orange juice," he replied.

I made a couple of suggestions, one of which was to eliminate the orange juice. Just one week later John shared with the class that when he avoided the orange juice, his energy level stayed constant. Because he had been consistently ingesting large amounts of high-glycemic foods, he had become so intolerant to glucose that when he drank the high-glycemic juice and ate cereals with refined sugars, he would crash. He needed to switch to a diet that was balanced with more low-glycemic foods.

Laura was forty years old, a working mom, and a wife. She had been steadily gaining weight over the past few years and could now accurately be called overweight. Besides that, she had absolutely no energy. She felt particularly tired around ten o'clock in the morning and three o'clock in the afternoon. She said she had been unable to lose weight.

Laura also experienced depression and she craved sweets. She definitely felt older than her age, was always tired, and was borderline diabetic. Laura's dietary analysis showed that she skipped breakfast, snacked on candy bars and cookies, drank up to ten cans of soda a day, and ate her largest meal at night.

Even though she was unaware of it, Laura was an expert at feeding the sugar monster that produced all the symptoms of her high-glycemic diet. Before she could possibly expect to lose a pound, she had to learn how to put the sugar monster to sleep.

> Before she could possibly expect to lose a pound, she had to learn how to put the sugar monster to sleep.

The key factor in doing this is remembering that every time we ingest fuel (food), a biochemical reaction takes place. In her case, the high-glycemic diet was inducing a hypoglycemic reaction. As Laura continued to eat these types of foods day in and day out, her pancreas was constantly being over stimulated. Consequently, she was creating too high an insulin response too often.

This caused her metabolism to slow down, which contributed to her weight gain. The over-stimulated insulin response caused by the simple sugars she ate regularly stole sugar from her blood, causing her to feel tired every day. And because of her lack of physical activity, the simple sugars or carbohydrates she was eating converted into stored fat.

You can imagine how frustrating it was for her. She was trying to lose weight, have more energy, and feel alive. But she was doing all the wrong things—things that prohibited weight loss and made her feel tired and depressed.

Laura came to our group fitness class, which consisted of three forty-five-minute exercise sessions a week. I outlined some basic dietary guidelines for her to follow that would serve as a starting point: eat low-glycemic foods that were compatible with her blood type; add protein to her meals; and have protein shakes between meals. I also suggested that she take a few dietary supplements on a regular basis. I knew if she would follow these few suggestions as best as she could, there was hope.

Laura herself took the biggest step of all. She got off the couch.

Two weeks later, when she entered the fitness class, Laura had a new glow to her skin and a sparkle in her eyes. She really looked fresh, healthier, and alive. Laura told me that her energy remained level throughout the day and that she felt better than she had in years. Now she had a clear mind and did not crave sugar.

If you want to gain better control of your sweet tooth, overcome those feelings of depression and sluggishness, and avoid potential serious health problems, then eliminate or minimize your simple sugars and replace them with low-glycemic or complex carbohydrates. These are the foods numbered from 0 to 50 on the glycemic index chart. Low-glycemic foods contain multi-chain molecules that burn more slowly, like a time-released food. They do not give a quick spike of insulin and immediate energy, but instead they promote an even insulin response and convert to energy over a longer period of time.

Switching from a simple sugar to a complex carbohydrate could simply mean choosing brown rice over white rice. You don't have to go without—just make some switches that will give you a steady energy level, less spiking in your insulin response, and more control over craving sweets. Plus, they will enhance your metabolic process.

Over the next few weeks Laura dropped pounds and inches, something she wasn't able to do before. Now her body was beginning to function the way it was originally designed to function. At last, it could perform optimally for her.

Once we get the machine in good operating order, the rest is a piece of cake!

Speaking of cake, there is nothing wrong with having those occasional goodies. The problems begin when they are the rule instead of the exception. If you walk by a dessert tray and feel like having something sweet, then go for it. But if you walk by that tray and it grabs you like a vice grip and says, "Eat me, or else," then the sugar monster is still wide awake in you. By eating lower glycemic foods, you can put the sugar monster to sleep forever.

Protein—Stimulus for Weight Loss

Just as carbohydrates stimulate an insulin response, protein stimulates another hormone named glucagon. Glucagon's function is the opposite of insulin's. Glucagon encourages the body to burn fats, stabilizes the blood sugar, strengthens the immune system, suppresses the appetite, and supports protein synthesis. When it is stimulated by protein, this hormone will cause the body to burn fat more readily, reduce hunger and cravings for sweets, and protect the immune system. It is responsible for aiding the body to maintain lean weight. If you are on a high-carbohydrate and low-protein diet, you can see why it will be virtually impossible to lose weight or fat. Your body needs adequate amounts of protein daily. As a rule, you should ingest 1 gram of protein for every 2.2 pounds of body weight. If you exercise regularly and are very physically active, then I would recommend 1 to 1.5 or more grams of protein per 2.2 pounds of body weight.

To stimulate weight loss, make sure your meals and snacks favor protein over carbohydrates. Eating a meal that has more protein calories than carbohydrate calories is considered to be an anabolic meal. Creating anabolic momentum will cause your body to burn fat for energy, thereby stabilizing blood sugar levels and supplying the muscle tissues with the nutrition they need to repair and build.

Should you choose to eat from the glycemic index and the protein chart, make sure your food selections are compatible to your blood type (that information is to follow). This will not feel like a diet. It will allow your body to function properly and will improve your digestive and immune system. It will become a way of life.

Protein Choices

Here are some protein-rich foods that you can choose from to go with your meals or snacks. All meats should be lean. Do not eat deli meats.

▶ Turkey and chicken

▶ Eggs, egg whites, or egg substitute

▶ Low-fat cottage cheese

▶ Low-fat yogurt

▶ Tofu

▶ Fish, broiled or baked

▶ Red meat

▶ Low-fat cheese

▶ Nuts

▶ Protein shakes

Staying Hydrated

Drinking enough water is critical to staying well. Try starting out with a glass of water every hour. Spike it with lemon or lime if that will help you to drink it. To find out the amount of water you should drink daily, convert one-half of your body weight to ounces. That's how many ounces of water you should drink daily. For example, if you weigh 150 pounds, you need 75 ounces of water a day.

Avoid or minimize sodas and fruit drinks, and avoid fruit juices made from concentrates. Herbal teas, particularly green tea, are better choices than coffee. Drinks with caffeine will contribute to dehydration, so it is best to avoid those, also.

Eating For Weight Management

The inclination to become fat or overweight is induced by lifestyles that lack physical activities and are full of poor food selections, including an abundance of processed and fast foods. We'll talk about the role exercise and being active in the Exercise section of the book. But for now, remember the rule of thumb for eating:

▸ Eat when you are hungry.
▸ Stop when you are satisfied (not stuffed).
▸ Don't eat if you are not hungry. You may be emotionally distraught instead of hungry.

Food nourishes our bodies, not our minds or our emotions. There is nothing on your plate that can meet your emotional needs. Regardless of your current feelings or the state of your emotions, do not allow this to cross over to your plate of food. Examine what your real motives are.

If you are anxious or tense, go for a walk or have a workout. If you are depressed or feeling unloved and not needed, call someone who will make you laugh. When you feel stressed, pray, meditate, and do relaxation exercises. When you are angry, forgive. When you are sad, hug someone. When you are tired, go to sleep.

The success of your journey (in addition to the dietary and exercise tools) includes the state of your emotions, your attitude, and how you manage them.

Pursue a balanced life!

— Renewing Your Mind —

() Certainly being overweight may significantly affect your health and well-being more than it does your appearance. As you set out to overcome the yo-yo diet dilemma by losing weight and keeping it off, do the potential health dangers serve as motivational reasons? Yes, or no? If no, review the connection with obesity and illness in this chapter. Maintaining a healthy weight will give you the luxury of enjoying a better quality of life. As you learn to keep your weight off for life, continue to remind yourself of your motivational reasons for pursuing your ideal weight.

() Many times individuals with sincere intentions need to re-evaluate the types of foods they eat because it is easy to get off course without even being aware of it. Does your diet consist of high-glycemic foods? Yes, or no? If yes, take time to review the listing of the samples of foods in this chapter. You will discover that weight management for the long haul requires a dietary checkup from time to time. Managing what food types you eat will help you manage your weight!

( ) Our attitude towards food plays a huge role in our being successful with weight management. You may have an attitude that hinders your ability to keep the weight off, like *I live to eat*. Do you live to eat? Yes, or no? If yes, then remember that you need to control food, not have food control you. Enjoy eating. Food has wonderful flavors, textures, and aromas. Enjoy the smells and flavors and textures, but remind yourself that food is for nourishment of your body. Nothing more! Food is a means to get you to where you are planning to go!

( ) See Appendix A for more information about protein shakes, meal replacements, supplements, and other nutritional food products.

As fire extinguished by an excess of fuel, so is the natural health of the body destroyed by an intemperate diet.

—*Burton*

Chapter

10

The Despair of Dieting

O H, NO!" CAME THE SCREAM FROM THE WARM-UP ROOM. My student and I looked at each other in surprise. Though we were training a room away, we still heard the shriek. Should we go to see what happened? Before we could decide, we heard the stationary bike going furiously. That sound brought knowing smiles to our lips as we realized what the scream of despair was all about.

At that time, I owned and operated several personal training and nutritional counseling studios. As students arrived, they went directly to the warm-up room to spend the first fifteen minutes biking to prepare for the thirty-minute circuit-training workout we would do together.

Both at the request of my students and for the purpose of calculating body fat percentages, I had put scales in the warm-up rooms.

Most students jumped onto the scale as soon as they entered to see if they were winning the battle—or to see how badly they were losing. The number on the scale had evoked that scream from Mary.

> Sadly, most people would rather swim in a pool of familiar ignorance by going on yet another diet than swim in an ocean of unfamiliar truths.

As soon I finished training my student, Mary came in to start her workout. I didn't mention her scream; however, as we started training, I asked how her weekend had gone. That was all it took for the tears to begin to flow.

Sadly, most people would rather swim in a pool of familiar ignorance by going on yet another diet than swim in an ocean of unfamiliar truths.

Overwhelmed by her guilt, Mary began confessing all her dietary sins to me. She told me how badly she had done over the weekend. She felt so guilty for eating foods she was "not allowed to eat." She wistfully told me how she had been doing good for a while on her diet, but then she fell off her diet and began to binge. After giving me a rundown of the foods she ate, she was nearly exhausted. I had to stop her in the middle of the workout to calm her down.

I wasn't completely shocked by her state of mind because the scream from the warm-up room was all too familiar. But, having once been a 305-pound doughboy myself, my heart went out to her. I understood her struggle to beat this weight problem, and I felt her pain of defeat.

So I gently reminded her of my philosophy—one that I believed would break this cycle of guilt and pain. "Mary, do you remember that I didn't teach you to **diet** to lose weight? So how could you have 'gone off' your diet?"

"I read about a diet in a ladies' magazine," she blurted out. "It guaranteed to drop several pounds in just a few days. So I started it, but I couldn't stay on it."

I knew her intentions were good and she was determined to succeed. But she, like so many others who are victimized by their own desperation, was easy prey for any information that offered a quick remedy to her problem. In Mary's case, her desperation put her in touch with the wrong approach to getting her weight under control—one that would not bring ultimate success.

It's sometimes frightening to think how many people live in fear and trembling when it comes to weight and diet. The emotional stresses that people feel when they go on a diet are totally unnecessary.

The scale means little when it comes to monitoring success of eating to lose weight. Weight management is multidimensional, and eating is just one aspect. Sadly, most people would rather swim in a pool of familiar ignorance of going on yet another diet than swim in an ocean of unfamiliar truths. For some, it must feel safer to stay within their comfort zones—to keep following the same ways that have over and over proved to be unsuccessful, somehow still retaining the hope that one day success will come. That is a true journey down the road to insanity.

A Trip to Diet Island

Let me take you on a journey to Diet Island, and I never expect you to have to go on this journey again! For now, just sit back and enjoy the cruise as this ship takes you away to an island where "going on a diet" is king.

The cruise begins on Friday night. As you step onto the cruise ship, you notice how well appointed it is. You are sure you are going to enjoy the ride to Diet Island. Somehow the atmosphere seems to promise that you will finally be happy, that soon you will feel good enough about yourself to lie on a white sand beach in a bikini.

Your thoughts are interrupted by the dinner bell, and boy, is dinner scrumptious! You don't want to miss a thing, so later you have the midnight snack even though you aren't hungry.

On Saturday morning you eat a full breakfast and enjoy walking on the deck. Then comes the barbecue on the promenade. Someone reminds you to stay up for the midnight dessert buffet; you don't have to be told twice.

On Sunday you skip breakfast and sleep in. The Sunday brunch, though, is worth getting up for. Then, after a lazy afternoon of lounging on the deck, you decide just to have dessert for dinner. But that doesn't really fill you up, so you go to the late-night buffet.

That's OK, you think. *I can handle this diet for awhile. It's only for a few weeks. Then I'll have the rest of my life to enjoy food again. The reward will be worth it.*

As you enjoy the ride back, your mind wanders back. You heard about your destination, Diet Island, from someone, somewhere, who told you how someone she knew went to this island and lost fifteen pounds in just ten days. You can't wait to have results like that. It will be worth the sacrifice.

Early Monday morning the island comes into view. You don't see any of the lush tropical vegetation and pristine beaches you expected. In fact, it looks like it's a desert island—mostly stretches of dry, hot sand with just a few scrawny weeds here and there. *That's OK,* you tell yourself. *I've finally made a commitment that once and for all I will be free of fat—no matter what.*

You will need to be taught how to go on a diet, so your new teacher meets you at the dock. Your teacher's name is Mr. Diet. Later, you find out from another visitor that his first name is "Going On A," but he doesn't like for people to know that.

After a quick drink of water (you wish it had been a cold soda), you are led to the introductory session. You find Mr. Diet inflexible and unforgiving. He reveals that all the information you will receive there is only good for the time that you are on the island. It's no good once you go back home.

That's OK, you tell yourself. *I'll have everything I need by the time I leave here.*

> That's OK, you think. I can handle this diet for awhile. It's only for a few weeks.

At this point Mr. Diet takes total control of your life. He lists the rules of behavior, which must be followed to the tee. Severe penalties await if you violate any. Plus, there is no leaving the island to have fun. You are not allowed to enjoy life or enjoy any food as long as you are on this island. And that is the way it will be for the duration.

That's OK, you think. *I can handle this diet for a while. It's only for a few weeks. Then I'll have the rest of my life to enjoy food again. The reward will be worth it.*

"It's uncertain how long you will spend on this island. It could be two or three weeks, a few months…or even the rest of your life. It all depends on your willpower," the teacher sternly informs you. A chill runs down your spine, but you ignore it.

After a full twelve-ounce glass of water and two carrots, your classroom instruction begins. You learn that eating is basically a system of punishment and reward. Your ability to muster up enough self-control to stay on your diet will determine how many rewards you receive. You must work diligently at using your willpower.

To ensure your success, you are constantly reminded and warned of the devastation that you will cause to yourself if for some reason you should go "off" your diet. Going off your diet is unacceptable, and there will be severe penalties applied, including guilt, frustration, and a personal sense of failure.

First, you must avoid any and all foods that you like or that taste good. "Nutritious can never be delicious." You have to memorize that and make it your mantra. You must learn how to sacrifice, go without, and accept deprivation as a virtue.

Second, you must learn to eat very few calories because calories are your worst enemy. You will become so familiar with your enemy on this island that you will know the exact number in their army no matter in which food they come hidden. If you lose count, you are told, they will overtake you and conquer you.

Hand in hand with counting calories comes starvation. You must learn the art of starvation and deprivation so that you don't go off your diet and commit the one cardinal dietary sin: **the binge**. This sin will cause such defeat that the teacher preaches against it for a long time.

That's OK, you tell yourself. *None of this really matters because I've been around long enough to know that dieting is the only way to lose weight.* So you're pumped and ready to suck it up. What's the big deal about going on a diet anyway? *You can do it.*

After reviewing your diet plan, Mr. Diet gives you the main tool for determining your success: a bathroom scale. Yes, now you are ready to begin the regimen.

The first thing that you do the next morning and every morning that follows is weigh yourself. For the first two weeks you see the scale reading less and less each day, and you are thrilled. You are beginning to feel good about yourself. In fact, you can almost look into the mirror without cringing. *Bikini, here I come!* You feel very positive that this time the diet is not going to let you down. It's actually working. You've cut back on your calories, you've learned how to starve and deprive yourself, you're going without…and you're dropping weight!

Then, after the first three weeks, something just isn't right. You feel tired all the time, and you're not as chipper as you were before. Plus, your weight has quit going down. It isn't going up, but it isn't going down, either. *How can this be happening?* You're doing everything Mr. Diet told you to do.

In a state of panic you decide to make some changes to your diet—covertly, of course. You cut back on calories because they are the enemy. That should fix the problem.

The next day, and the next you go back to the scale for the reward, but no weight has been lost. *What's wrong?* Now you feel a sense of urgency, almost panic. Every morning, noon, and night you weigh yourself to look for your reward. *All this sacrificing to no avail?* Impossible! But the scale is not changing. You have stopped dropping weight.

Not only has the scale become unfriendly, but you feel worse than ever. You're terribly grumpy and irritable, and nobody can come near you. You feel less and less able to cope with the lack of nutrition, and what's worse—*you're hungry*. You are so hungry that you can't think of anything but all those good-tasting foods that your teacher said you must sacrifice. The cravings are driving you crazy.

You recognize these horrifying warning signs, those signs that signal the attack of the dietary cardinal sin. But you can no longer help yourself. You fought it the best you could, and your will-power is gone. Your determination and desire have been overcome by weakness and hunger. All your effort and sacrifice are a thing of the past. You are out of control and you are ready to binge.

You stow away on the next ship that leaves, which just happens to be a cargo ship that is bringing vegetables to the island, and as soon as you arrive on land, you race to the first fast-food place, ice cream stand, or doughnut shop that you spot. You are completely out of control, and the cravings for sugar are so strong that you would kill for something sweet.

The cruise is over, the island adventure is shot, your pocketbook is smaller, and your diet has turned out to be your enemy. Once again, you've become frustrated, discouraged, and more depressed than before you went to the island. Over the next couple of weeks, the weight comes back on, and you wonder how many extra pounds it will take before you drum up enough willpower to return to Diet Island again.

Freedom from Dieting

If you have been around the last twenty years or so, I'm certain you have visited Diet Island once or twice. That's because dieting has become a way of life for many. If you have been to Diet Island, there is a good chance that you are included somewhere in the following statistics:

▸   More than one in five children ages six through seventeen are overweight.
▸   Thirty-two million American women between the ages of twenty and seventy-four are overweight.
▸   Americans spend nearly ten billion per year on diet aids.

- In 1998, twenty-seven percent of U.S. adults were currently dieting.
- Only five percent of all dieters will have maintained their weight loss.

The quick-fix approach to losing weight will not bring you success, and its effects on your health and appearance will not be positive. If you have dieted before, then you have probably experienced the drudgery of a weight-loss diet, and how unrealistic sticking to it can be.

Learning the difference between going on a weight-loss diet and eating a healthy, well-balanced diet is the first step toward long-term success.

It's great to be known as a person who has a lot of willpower, but willpower is not the key that unlocks the door to dietary freedom. Neither is starvation or deprivation. Starving or depriving yourself is outdated, physiologically inaccurate, and should never be a part of your life again. This type of approach to dieting is directly responsible for maintaining body fat. Your dieting efforts have most likely proven one basic truth: Weight loss from dieting is temporary (at best) and makes your body fatter than when you started the diet.

When I conduct seminars on weight management and diets, my favorite question for my audience is, "How many of you have ever gone on a diet to lose weight?" Usually, about eighty-five percent of the people raise their hands. Then I ask the next question, "How many of you lost weight?" About sixty percent respond positively. Then I asked the big one, "How many of you who lost weight on your weight-loss diets have gained it back again?" Just about ninety-five percent of them indicate they have.

What does that say about dieting? Did they fail, did the diet plan fail, or is the idea of dieting a failure?

My goal is to set you free from the bondage of dieting by raising your awareness of what dieting *is* and what dieting *is not*. You will learn that you are free to enjoy food without the sense of guilt that so often accompanies the dieting mentality. You will be set free from the yo-yo syndrome and the fear of going off your diet.

> What does that say about dieting? Did they fail, did the diet plan fail, or is the idea of dieting a failure?

That's why the information in this section will not lead you to go on a diet. You will experience dietary freedom for the first time in your life while at the same time maintain a healthy body weight. You will be able to have a potentially disease-free life, one that is full of energy. The frustration, self-inflicted stress, and the tremendous sense of failure associated with dieting to lose weight will become a thing of the past. You will embark on perhaps a brand new approach to eating that will literally set you free from the bondage of dieting.

Blood Type / Diet Connection
Something Is Wrong

For the greater part of my life I have been a fairly healthy person. But sometime in 1986 I felt my health was going downhill. I was losing the ability to function normally on a day-to-day basis. I wasn't sure what was wrong, but it was like having to endure a nightmare during the day.

Every day around ten in the morning and three in the afternoon, I would crash. I could actually roll over and fall asleep in the middle of a training session, business meeting or while driving my car. I realized that I had been experiencing these symptoms for about five years, but they were getting worse.

At the time, I was buried in my personal training business, which required long days, most of my energy and time, plus all the stress I could handle. For lunch I would usually sneak out for some Chinese food. Then I would go back to the studio.

Immediately after I ate I had tons of energy and felt great, but within an hour or so, my energy dropped like a roller coaster. I would be in the middle of a training session with a client, and yet I could hardly keep my eyes open. Not only was I tired and sleepy, but many times I would feel anxious, light-headed, and lethargic. Mentally I was experiencing brain fog. I even had the feeling of being depressed, for no reason.

One evening in 1986, Lori and I were out for a drive. We had splurged on a couple of candy bars, the all-American health snack. I needed to gas up the car, so I pulled into the service station. However, when I tried to get out of the car to pump the gas, I just couldn't because I felt so weak. I had to ask Lori to pump the gas because I could not keep my eyes open a moment longer. It was just as if I was poisoned. By the time she got back into the car, I had passed out at the wheel.

That incident led me to see a doctor for some tests, including a glucose test, which came out positive. My results from the glucose test showed that I was hypoglycemic, or that I had low blood sugar. Hypoglycemia, or low blood sugar, occurs when blood levels of glucose (a form of sugar that is the body's main fuel) drops too low to fuel the body's activity. This is generally due to over-stimulating the pancreas by eating the wrong carbohydrates and too many too often, causing an over-insulin response. An over abundance of insulin robs the blood of the sugar and the individual feels a loss of energy or crashing affect. The symptoms of hypoglycemia can include drowsiness, weakness, dizziness, hunger and confusion. At times headache, irritability, trembling, rapid heartbeat, sweating and a cold, clammy feeling may also be symptoms. In severe cases, a person may lose consciousness or even lapse into a coma.

I was given some material to read and a list of foods: *forbidden* and *permissible*. Can you imagine having to live that way? That just wasn't acceptable to me. I promised myself that I would find another way to correct this debilitating condition.

In the meantime, I followed the list, but eating the prescribed foods didn't give me much relief. The physician advised me to incorporate some milk for a protein source, which would slow down the insulin response. He also suggested that I eat wheat bread. Still, adding those two foods did not help.

I struggled for another ten years and I decided that if I had to live like that for the rest of my life, I would dread living. How horrible life can be when your health is upside down!

This condition prompted me to research and to experiment personally. First, because I was familiar with the use of the glycemic index for making food selections, I began to follow this plan of eating low glycemic foods for a while because I thought it would help me to control my blood sugar. I did start to feel a little change for the better. My blood sugar seemed to level out more often than before, but I was still struggling every day to stay awake and alert and I was still experiencing the loss of energy.

It All Made Sense

Having been introduced to some studies and reading a book suggested to me by my brother about one's genetics and the link between an individual's blood type and what foods to eat, I recognized the puzzle pieces. Later, I involved myself in additional studies and research that showed the link between blood type, diet and disease, illness, and longevity. I began conducting focus groups, body redesigning sessions based on one's genetic individuality and weight loss. Because the theory is based strictly on one's genetics and not on mainstream dietary practices, this supported what I always believed: One diet does **not** fit all!

The missing link in today's world of dietary practices is the factoring in of one's genetic individuality. The approach to making food selections has always been a one-diet-fits-all concept. The one-diet-for-everyone is a common mentality used by most dieticians, nutritionists, and the average health care practitioner.

More and more studies and research on how one's DNA, genetics, and genetic individuality are being conducted. Results from the new findings will provide accuracy for determining and treating potential illnesses from those in the medical community. More natural health practitioners are also moving in that direction. The fact that specialized diets are given to heart patients, diabetics, and people with various other illnesses and diseases shows some improvement. But these professionals still haven't seemed to make the connection that *one diet doesn't suit every person*. A diet plan that suggests that it will work for everyone is ludicrous and old school…and it should send up a red flag for you if it is suggested to you as a way to lose weight.

Your goal is not to lose weight for a short period of time and regain it. Your goal is keeping that weight off with the least amount of effort—for life!

I determined which foods were most compatible for my blood type and which were actually toxic for my blood type. Then, I made the appropriate dietary adjustments.

When I did, something happened to me that I hadn't experienced in about fifteen years. Besides my body immediately losing body fat and increasing muscularity, I no longer experienced the gas and bloating that used to be normal after I had eaten a meal. I had thought this was normal! Plus, I had constant energy throughout the entire day. The brain fog was gone. Finally, no more crashing! After all the months and years I spent wasting my time, it only took about eight days of eating correctly for my blood type to allow my blood sugar to stabilize. My blood sugar has remained stable ever since.

Eating correctly for your blood type is the *stay power* for you to reach your ideal weight, keep it, and enjoy a healthier, more energetic, and disease-free life.

The Exciting Results

My blood type is O. I am genetically designed to be a red meat eater as my primary source of protein. That might sound alarming to you because it goes against the current thinking that red meat is an unhealthy source of protein. But that is not true, especially for people with type O blood.

Before I started eating this way, I had red meat maybe once a month. But as soon as I realized that individuals with O blood types are genetically compatible for digesting, assimilating, and utilizing red meat, I decided to eat it more often. I decided that if I were going to benefit from this relatively new concept, I would have to give a hundred percent effort. So I did.

For the first six months I ate approximately one to two pounds of red meat daily as my primary source of protein. (My preference is free-range meat, but that is not always practical.) The meat should be lean as possible. I also ate plenty of vegetables and fruits that were compatible for my type. Additionally, I avoided foods that were not compatible at least 90% of the time, including junk foods.

Here was a typical day of what I ate:

Breakfast (one of the following):

- One to three eggs, a petite steak, and peppermint tea
- One to two slices of toasted Ezekiel (made from sprouted grain) or millet bread with butter or almond nut butter and organic black cherry jam and peppermint tea
- One chocolate protein shake (w/compatible protein powder) w/ soy or almond milk or water (my grab-and-go breakfast)
- Sparkling water was my in between meals drink until later drinking mainly alkaline water. I took supplements every morning, also.

Mid-morning snack (one of the following):

- Handful of walnuts and pitted prunes
- Chocolate protein-shake or protein bar
- Handful of semi-sweet chocolate chips and almonds

Lunch:

- Caesar salad (without the dressing), liver, and broccoli.
- An 8-ounce petite sirloin with broccoli, a sweet potato, and a salad
- Chocolate protein shake

My mid-afternoon snack:

- Same as my morning snack

Evening meal:

▶ Similar to my lunch, sometimes substituting fish for steak

▶ Fresh mixed salads with veggies with all meals.

▶ If I felt hungry in the evening, I'd drink a chocolate protein shake. (See Appendix A.)

At the end of those six months I thought it wise to get some blood work done and see how my body was reacting to this new way of eating. The outside was looking good, but I needed a look at the inside.

When I got my blood work results back I was elated! My total cholesterol was down from 180 to 150, my HDL (good cholesterol) read 49, my LDL (bad cholesterol) read 87, and my triglycerides were 68.

What did all that mean? Simply put, after adding red meat to my diet as a staple protein source for six months and avoiding foods that were incompatible to my blood type, my blood work showed me that my blood lipids were in the low-normal ranges. That meant that (contrary to current opinion) my intake of animal protein did not induce elevated cholesterol levels. In fact, it contributed to lowering them. Astonishing? Not for a type O! Does that mean everyone should eat red meat as a primary source of protein? No, but we type O people can.

By knowing more about your genetic individuality, you will eventually experience that dietary freedom exists when you factor in your genetics into your eating patterns. And the best part is you can say *goodbye to dieting* and *hello to Instinctive Eating.*

— Renewing Your Mind —

() The despair of dieting is such an unnecessary experience. Have you been one who has tried more than one diet to lose weight, only to have a Diet Island experience? Yes, or no? If yes, then by now you are either totally ready to give up or are still hoping there is a diet that will work for you. Remember the diet is only a part of the obesity or overweight solution. By understanding that food is a source of fuel for your body it is best to learn which foods are best for you. Eating doesn't mean being "good" or "bad," or going on and off a diet. Eating is something you should feel free to do with out the element of guilt or failure.

() Changing your mind-set or way of thinking about food may seem a bit foreign If it has been a negative experience in the past. Weight loss and diet go hand in hand, but not dieting the weight off. If you have been victimized by a Diet Island experience, just remember this: eating food shouldn't have to be a learned behavior. *Why* you make certain food selections has to be learned. Eating food should be a lifestyle-friendly experience whether for losing weight, maintaining weight, or even gaining weight. Dieting doesn't allow for this!

The most natural and individualized way to make food selections a reality for life is by listening to your body's responses.

—Dr. Joe

Chapter

11

Instinctive Eating

W HEN WE EAT, BIOCHEMICAL RESPONSES TO THE FOODS WE ingest occur within our bodies. These specific reactions and responses are a part of our natural biological design. The way our bodies react to particular foods is the most accurate monitoring tool we can use for losing weight, improving energy, stabilizing blood sugar, controlling cholesterol levels, and defeating a host of other health-related disorders that interfere with our ability to lead healthy and energetic lives. Learning to listen to our body's responses to what we ingest and making food selections that are positive for us is what I refer to as *Instinctive Eating*.

If we were like the animals in the animal kingdom, we would not have all the health-related problems associated with the foods we eat. Consider the lion for a moment. No one has to tell a lion to eat red meat, and you would never catch a lion climbing a banana tree for bananas. How about the horse? He doesn't gravitate to red meat but rather oats, grains, and grass. Why? Animals eat instinctively. It is their mechanism for survival. Not so for humans. Our food choices are usually prompted by social gatherings, ethnic and family traditions, religious rules, emotions, and even food advertisements—to name just a few. In general, you name it and we'll eat it.

We have gotten so out of touch with eating properly that we have adapted the reward/punishment system for selecting our nutrition. We mostly base our food selections on our emotional states at the moment. Healthy food choices are often correlated to a form of sacrifice and punishment; junk food is a reward for being good. Just ask your kids!

Eating food has nothing to do with being *good* or *bad*—at least it shouldn't. If you have made yourself a victim of self-imposed punishment for not eating healthily or for not sticking to your diet, then STOP! Eating food is a means of fueling our bodies. The biochemical reactions induced by the foods you eat are directly connected to your own genetic predisposition or makeup. It's like knowing the difference between whether you are pumping diesel fuel for a diesel engine, or gasoline for a gas engine—the consequences can be serious if you mix them up, just as the consequences can be serious for your health if you are not making correct food selections for your blood type.

Becoming aware of how your body reacts to food is the first place to start. You have to teach yourself to listen to your body. Let your body, **not** a diet plan, be your teacher.

Listen to Your Body

If you were genetically wired so that every time you ingested something that was not compatible with your chemistry or blood type you became violently ill, you might become an instinctive eater in a hurry. Our bodies do have specific responses to different foods. Though not usually violent, most of us are not listening to the more subtle ways our bodies respond.

The beauty of eating correctly for one's blood type is that the biochemical reactions and responses to the foods we ingest allow our body to become our dietary teacher. We just have to pay attention to it. This approach to eating allows our bodies to do the talking. I'll show you how to listen.

Because I am Italian, I used to eat pasta, tomato sauce, and black pepper four to five times a week. Following the meal I had heartburn, gas, and bloating. Now if that wasn't a negative reaction, I don't what was! But I wasn't paying attention to my body's responses with respect to whether the food I just ate was compatible or not because I wasn't aware of the association of food with blood type. It was "normal" for me to feel that way after eating pasta—but not healthy. So I would do like most people and take a spoonful of some pink stuff to put out the fire in my chest.

When I made the connection between my body's responses to the food I ate, I became an instinctive eater. Biochemical reactions such as these prove beyond a shadow of a doubt that everyone is not the same. Proper food selection is vitally important. Awareness to these responses will promote instinctive eating, the most natural and individualized way to make food selections.

When I avoided the foods that were not compatible with my blood type, not only did the heartburn disappear, but so did the gas and the bloating. My body composition improved and I became more muscular, plus my blood sugar remained stable after all those previous miserable experiences of crashing.

Not all *Avoid Foods* (see list in the next chapter) cause negative reactions that are crippling or disruptive. Some incompatible foods contribute to illness and disease without any notice—sort of like laying a baseline for damaging your future health profile. But most incompatible foods will give you negative signs or symptoms if you learn to pay attention to your body. They can be as mild as gas, bloating, or diarrhea or more severe like acid reflux, intestinal discomfort, or gastrointestinal pain. They can be dangerous by increasing blood cholesterol levels, causing arthritic-like pain in the joints, colon toxicity, excess body fat, elevated blood pressure, liver and kidney dysfunction, and others.

The more you adhere to eating correctly for your blood type, the more dramatic your body's functionality improves. Conversely, the negative responses become elevated when you choose to eat the incompatible or *Avoid Foods* for your blood type. Foods that are incompatible to your blood type are not what are generally considered junk foods like potato chips, candy, and desserts. In many cases the food staples that you have learned to love and think are healthy may be incompatible to your body. Some of these may contribute to elevated cholesterol, while others slow your metabolism and interfere with your body's ability to lose weight. Incompatible foods can cause low blood sugar and hypoglycemia (a precursor to diabetes) as well as gas, bloating, indigestion, and irritable bowel syndrome.

Instead of following the trend of taking medicine for those dietary symptoms, start listening to your body and avoid the foods that are contributing to the problems.

Natural Detoxification

When you consume foods that are not compatible with your individual body type, your body can become toxic. Toxicity can occur in tissue, particularly fatty tissue, but also in the blood, the joints, and organs. By eating compatible foods and avoiding the incompatible ones (instinctive eating), your body actually undergoes a detoxification. Your bodily systems—the digestive system, colon, kidneys, liver, and the immune system—begin to operate as they were designed to. After the body adjusts to the compatible foods, an improvement in bodily function and performance follows. With improved bodily functions from the body's ridding itself of the toxins stored in the fat cells, the result is often weight loss.

Natural Weight Loss

Compatible (*Beneficial/Neutral*) and incompatible (*Avoid*) foods affect weight loss differently. Say, for example, a blood type O person needs to lose excess fat and includes food made from wheat in his diet, thinking that wheat products are healthy.

His body begins its response, but the response is not what was anticipated. The response is actually the opposite of the intended goal. Because all wheat products (other than sprouted wheat) are not compatible for the O blood type, the individual's metabolic system is challenged and losing weight is very difficult. The problem occurs at the cell's insulin receptors which prohibit the body from breaking down and releasing the carbohydrates properly, so weight loss in prohibited. Additionally the digestive system cannot function properly, which makes proper digestibility and assimilation nearly impossible. This all changes when compatible foods for the blood type are ingested. The bodily functions improve and the machine parts are working as they were designed to for that blood type.

One of the many benefits from making food selections that are compatible to your blood type is losing body fat. It takes all the work out of trying to lose weight by going on a weight loss diet. Since your body has been designed to carrying a natural or ideal weight, all you have to do is make certain you are doing what needs to be done so that the bodily systems and functions are normalized. By avoiding the incompatible foods from your diet, the toxins once stored in the fat cells will dissipate and cause the fat cells to shrink.

Your body will always work towards reaching its ideal weight. If you continue eating this way, eventually you will reach your ideal weight and keep it for life. I am living proof.

— Renewing Your Mind —

◊ The preferred choice by most overweight individuals for losing weight is going on a weight loss diet plan, which has only proven to produce temporary results at best. A more lifestyle-friendly approach to eating that can be done for life is long overdue. How do you make your food selections—based upon what you want, or upon how you feel after you have eaten a certain food? You will learn more about eating for your blood type in the next chapter, but ultimately you want make food selections freely without the dependency of a diet program to do it for you. As you eat differently, look for positive changes in your current weight and health status. How you feel you will sharpen your ability to listen to your body. Look for:

- Improved digestive system—i.e., elimination of gas, bloating, and abdominal pain.
- Improved energy and stabilized blood sugar levels.
- Lower blood pressure and cholesterol readings.
- Weight loss.

◊ Give instinctive eating the acid test and see how you feel. Read on to see how you can make better food selections based upon your individuality.

Nobody can be exactly like me. Sometimes even I have trouble doing it.

—Tallulah Bankhead, Actress

Chapter

12

Your Individuality Can Fix the Problem

IN MY PERSONAL AND PROFESSIONAL EXPERIENCE OF MANAGING my weight for all these years, it has been learning who I am and identifying with my individuality that has been the "stay power" for lifelong results. This is the solution to avoiding excessive weight gain, losing weight, and not regaining it. Obesity and being overweight is not caused solely by what you and I eat (as we learned from the previous chapters) but is only a one of the dynamics of the problem. Therefore addressing the whole person and not just what they eat is necessary to fix the problem.

To fix the obesity and overweight problem facing the American population and those in other nations we must address the whole person. The problem is community wide and therefore there needs a community-wide mentality to fix it. Individuality makes one unique from the next person, but all people are also a part of the whole. When one's individuality is unknown, it has no value to the person themselves or to the whole. Knowing what and who you are lets you begin to solve the problem.

When identified and applied to the whole, your individuality will make the whole much better, but it can become your enemy if it becomes an issue of individualism. Individualism is always looking out for number one! It has a self-centered mind-set, always takes, and never gives. So as we better understand our individuality, not only will we benefit but so will the whole as it receives the best from each individual.

If you and I want to fix the problem of obesity and being overweight that has grown to a national and even global epidemic monster, then you and I need to zoom in on our individuality. It will take each of us starting with ourselves before there is something to contribute to the whole!

> The more you learn about yourself in body, mind, and spirit the greater the likelihood of acquiring the "stay power" for lifelong success after you lose weight.

Individuality and Tools

Your willingness to develop the **Never Go Back** attitude, identifying the emotional/food triggers that affect your decision making process, and your specific genetic characteristics for diet and exercise are the tools you need to work with to be successful for the long haul. The more you learn about yourself in body, mind, and spirit the greater the likelihood of acquiring the "stay power" for lifelong success after you lose weight.

Blood Type Characteristics and Food

Since we all must fuel our bodies (eat), let's peek at the premise behind linking our genetic individuality (blood type) and unique characteristics to the foods we select.

Why your blood type and food? "You are what you eat," or so it is said! But in this mind-set of genetic individuality it is better to say, "Eat what you are!" Each of us is bio-chemically designed to eat foods that are most compatible to our blood types. This is the theory for making food selections that I have been following for over ten years.

We begin to get an understanding of this important concept by taking a look at the animal kingdom. Animals like the lion are meat eaters. They know what to eat, as it is instinctive to them. Horses, on the other hand, know to eat oats and grass and are not big on meats. Why? It is instinct for survival.

Each blood type has different characteristics that allow it to eat, digest, and assimilate food best for that particular group. The blood type O individual is blessed with strong stomach acid production and powerful enzymes that can metabolize almost anything, meats in particular. Not so for the A, B, and AB blood types. Their digestibility and assimilation process is not as stout as the O, and they will face some consequences from their food selections.

What happens when we eat foods that are not compatible with our blood types? What consequences are there? Agglutination of the red blood cells occur. Here's how it works:

Your body protects itself from uninvited guests or invaders by producing antibodies. Your immune system produces all kinds of antibodies to protect you from foreign substances. Each antibody is designed to attach itself to a foreign substance or antigen. When your body recognizes an intruder, it naturally produces more antibodies to attack and destroy the intruder. The antibody then attaches, or "glues" itself, a phenomenon referred to as "agglutination." This is a basic picture of how your body does the protection work on your behalf at the cellular level without your having to do much.

This agglutination also occurs when you and I eat a particular food from a food group that is not compatible with our blood types. It can take place in the gut wall, liver, joints, brain, and in the blood—anywhere! The gluing of the red blood cells in a particular system, organ, or place in the body groups or clumps the red blood cells together and the clumping breaks down the functionality of that system or bodily function. You and I can recognize it (if we listen to our bodies) in the form of some symptom. When undetected for too long this condition will ultimately contribute to some form of disease, illness, or poor health condition. It will also slow down your body's ability to burn calories—not a good condition if you need to lose weight or want to keep it off.

In the food groups list for each blood type you will see that certain foods are categorized as *Avoid* foods. These are not junk foods. They are to be avoided because of the dietary protein lectin or molecule that causes the gluing effect found in those foods and the potential damaging affect they can have on tissue. It is the dietary lectins that glue themselves to the surface of the red blood cells, which, in turn, cause a clumping of the cells until a particular system malfunctions.

Making food selections that are compatible to your blood type and avoiding those which are not is not at all like going on a diet. It is a matter of applying your intelligence and genetic individuality into selecting the correct fuel for your particular machine. Let's check out some of the characteristics listed below that are unique with each blood type and see if you can't identify with what you are.

Blood Type A

Blood type A individuals typically have the thickest blood of all four types. Because of their predetermined blood viscosity, they must avoid certain foods. Unfortunately in America meat and potatoes have always been the staple food on every dinner table from coast to coast. And when you consider forty percent of the population are A blood type, people need to think about what foods they are commonly eating, especially if they are an A. Remember, A individuals have thick blood and due to the fact that they do not break down red meat very easily it tends not to digest well in the colon, causing colon toxicity and contributing to elevated cholesterol. As the lectins in the red meat glue themselves to red cells the blood tends to thicken and becomes stickier. The heart then has to pump harder, potentially causing high blood pressure, hypertension, and heart disease. This contributes to why type A individuals have the shortest life spans.

Another characteristic of A individuals is the low stomach acid production which is necessary for proper metabolic process and digestibility. Most type As will say they either do not care for red meat or when they eat it, they feel sluggish or it upsets their stomachs.

A constant diet of mainly meats and potatoes provides fewer nutrients, lowers immune function, and thickens the blood, leading to heart disease, cancer, and early death. That is why blood type A individuals are susceptible to heart disease and cancers.

The foods most harmful to type As in the long run are meat and dairy. The elimination of these two food groups will allow type A individuals the greatest potential to avoid heart disease and cancer. Tofu, soy products, unsalted red skin peanuts, red wine, and green tea are especially good for type As because they help fight cancer. Type As typically have lost the ability to make pepsin, a protein-digesting enzyme. Therefore, a more vegetarian diet or one of less dense protein products such as chicken, turkey, and Cornish hens is more easily digestible for As. Whole grains such as quinoa, millet, brown rice, and wild rice are preferable over wheat products due to over-sensitivity to such products.

Strengths:

▸ Adapts well to dietary and environmental changes

Weakness:

▶ Thick blood
▶ Shortest life spans
▶ Affected by stress more than other blood types
▶ Sensitive digestive tract
▶ Vulnerable immune system
▶ Inability to digest animal meat properly

Health Risks:

▶ Heart disease
▶ Cancer
▶ High blood pressure
▶ Hypertension
▶ Enlarged heart muscle
▶ Anemia
▶ Liver disorders
▶ Diabetes

Nutritional Profile:

▶ **Beneficial:** Soy beans, tofu, and green tea for anti-oxidant qualities; grouper, cod, and salmon; soy cheese and soy milk; lentils; broccoli, carrots, romaine lettuce, and spinach; blueberries, blackberries, cranberries, prunes, and raisins.

▶ **Avoid:** animal fats, meat and dairy products; potatoes; kidney, lima, and navy beans; wheat; eggplant, peppers, and tomatoes; cantaloupe and honeydew melons.

Blood Type B

The B blood types have the most flexible diets of all the types. They can eat some red meat as protein sources and they can assimilate milk and/or dairy products well, unlike their blood type A and O neighbors. They have a thin blood (similar to type Os) so they need not be overly concerned about heart disease.

Type B individuals would do best to eliminate all wheat, corn, tomatoes, peanuts and especially chicken from their diets. They can eat and readily digest a wide range of foods. Type B blood types can tolerate dairy products in moderation. Fermented dairy products like yogurt, Kefir, and cottage cheese would be the best for the B.

Moderation is the key word for the blood type B, who can handle a little bit of everything but should not overdo it on any single food.

Type Bs have the second longest life spans to that of the O. They seem to become muscular easily as they gain the benefits from eating red meat and its enormous amounts of the nutrients, B vitamins, and amino acids. They have difficulty with chicken meat as it (along with other incompatible foods for this type) contributes to potential autoimmune diseases.

Strengths:

▸ Naturally strong immune system
▸ Receives maximum nutrients from diet more than the A or AB

▸ Muscle development comes easier than the A or AB

Weakness:

▸ Skin disorders
▸ Foot problems

Health Risks:

▸ Polio
▸ Lupus
▸ Lou Gehrig's Disease
▸ Multiple sclerosis

Nutritional Profile:

▸ Eat meat in moderation
▸ Utilizes dairy products well
▸ **Beneficial:** lamb and venison; cod and grouper; farmer, Feta, and mozzarella cheese; kidney, lima, navy, and soy beans; broccoli, collard, and mustard greens; pineapples and plums.
▸ **Avoid:** chicken; American cheese and ice cream; wheat and white and yellow corn; pumpkin, tofu, persimmons, and rhubarb.

Blood Type AB

Blood type AB has both dominant genes and is known as the universal receiver.

ABs have the intolerances of the A blood types and the benefits of the B. They may be more prone to cancer, heart disease, and autoimmune diseases. There seems to be a clear indication for women of this blood type to have many menstrual problems—excessive bleeding, clotting, cramping, and irregular menstrual cycles. There is a clear pattern of hormonal imbalances with this type.

This is the rarest blood type and sometimes identified as the modern blood type. AB blood type individuals are very rare, making up less than four percent of the American population. Their single worst food is chicken. Like the blood type B, type ABs are negatively affected by chicken meat. Chicken contains a dietary lectin that is dangerous to them that may agglutinate (clot) the blood and may also lead to heart disease, cancer, and/or a host of other digestive and intestinal tract illnesses. Tofu, soy products, salted red skin peanuts, red wine, and green tea are especially good for type AB individuals because the antioxidant content found in the them help fight cancer and heart disease. Most dairy products can be tolerated in moderation.

ABs seem to become more muscular than the A types, but not easily as the B. ABs may do well by adding dietary supplementation to their diets and getting their proteins, amino acids, etc. from vegetable sources. Eating compatible meats in moderation is OK for this type.

Strengths:

▸ Two dominant gene traits
▸ Friendliest of all immune systems

Weaknesses:

▸ Pattern of hormonal imbalances
▸ Tendency to chemical imbalance disorders

Health Risks:

▸ Cancer
▸ Heart disease
▸ Anemia
▸ Autoimmune disease
▸ Menstrual disorders

Nutritional Profile:

▸ Limited to small amounts of animal protein
▸ **Beneficial:** turkey; cod and mahi-mahi; navy, pinto, and soy beans; oat and rice flour; collard, dandelion, and mustard greens; figs, grapes, and plums.
▸ **Avoid:** chicken; duck; all pork and venison; clams, crab, haddock, lobster, and shrimp; kidney and lima beans; white and yellow corn and peppers; guava, mangoes, and oranges.

Blood Type O

Blood type O individuals have thin blood, a strong immune system, produce abundant stomach acid, and have the longest life spans at present. Type O appears to be close to being the oldest blood type.

Both dairy and grains should be avoided. Most blood type O people are lactose intolerant. Soy milk and soy cheeses are the easiest and most tasty ways of replacing those much-loved dairy products. Os have a greater predisposition to celiac/sprue disease, which is the inability to digest gluten. Type O individuals who adhere to eating lean protein tend to have very low cholesterol levels and stay quite healthy.

Type O individuals digest red meat very well and it contributes to lowering their cholesterol levels and aids them in losing body fat. The O does not do well with dairy, wheat, nuts, or grains.

Plenty of vegetables, fruits, and protein from most all animals work best for the O. Wheat products appear to contribute to joint pain and arthritic-like discomfort. Many athletes are blood type O, as are many bodybuilders.

Because the O is very resilient and even can abuse their physiology for some time with no major problems, they tend to have the longest life spans. Due to their thin blood, type Os appear to be less problematic with plaque buildup in the arteries and have fewer chances of heart disease—at least early in life.

Strengths:

▸ Thinnest blood
▸ Strongest immune system
▸ Strongest stomach acid production
▸ Longest life span
▸ Metabolizes food very well
▸ Neutralizes cholesterol
▸ Low clotting risk

Weaknesses:

▸ Lacks blood clotting factor
▸ Intolerant to dairy and environmental conditions
▸ Most resilient to alcohol, smoking, etc.

Health risks:

▸ Strokes—due to clotting factor
▸ Blood disorders like hemophilia and leukemia
▸ Arthritis and/or inflammatory diseases
▸ Peptic ulcers
▸ Allergies

Nutritional Profile:

▸ Foods rich in vitamin K
▸ **Beneficial:** beef—primary source for protein; salmon; mozzarella cheese; pinto beans; artichoke, broccoli, and greens; figs and plums.

▶ **Avoid:** pork; wheat; corn; lentils and navy beans; cabbage, Brussels sprouts and white and red potatoes; melons and oranges.

Remember: the "stay power" to managing your weight for the rest of your life will have everything to do with factoring in your genetic individuality. But knowing the difference between the ideal world and the real world of food, I have always insisted on using my 80/20 rule when you are making food selections for your blood type. By eating 80% of your food selections for your blood type you will maximize the results you are looking for while still having the flexibility to eat 20% of the foods that are not compatible without interfering with your health or your progress. Eating has to be a way of life. (See Appendix A for more information about your blood type.)

— Renewing Your Mind —

◊ Do you know what blood type you are? Yes, or no? If no, one excellent way to find out is by donating blood at your local Red Cross! Not only will you be doing a great thing that may help save a life, but at the same time you'll find out what blood type you are. You may check with your doctor's office, but generally it is not kept on file. If you don't want to (or can't) give blood, there are home blood typing kits available. (See www. bodyredesigning.com.) Once you know your blood type you can take advantage of the information in this book as well as the in-depth information in any of the books listed in appendix A.

◯ As a nation of people, we have been programmed to accept mainstream thinking when it comes to diets, nutrition, and even exercise—that one-fits-all mentality. As history has proven, we have failed. But as you are learning more about yourself and your individuality, it starts to become very clear that everyone is not the same. What they eat should not be the same, either. Do you know the difference between plain junk foods and AVOID foods for your blood type? Yes, or no? If no, then here comes something to satisfy your taste buds. In my opinion, "junk" foods such as candies, chips, and other refined sugary products are not really foods at all, so they don't factor into this message. AVOID foods are the foods that may be good for one blood type but not good for you because of your individual blood type. Foods that are not compatible with your chemistry should be avoided. Become familiar with these and learn to choose other foods instead from the beneficial list for your type. And don't forget the 80/20% rule always applies!

Section IV: Exercise

Body Genetics

Those who think they have not time for bodily exercise will sooner or later have to find time for illness

—Edward Stanley

Chapter

13

Your Benefits Package

THE RETURN YOU GET FOR EXERCISING IS JUST LIKE THE benefits package you receive at your place of employment. You start off with a basic package, but over time you receive more benefits for staying with the company. Likewise, the longer you make exercise a part of your life, the better the benefits package gets. The beauty of exercising is you get all the physiological and health benefits, plus the emotional and psychological benefits that come from taking control of your life.

Before we examine the many benefits that await you, let me congratulate you on the wise decision you have made to develop a new attitude, emotional fortitude, physical fitness, and an improved wellness condition so you will **Never Go Back** to your former overweight condition again. You will never again allow the status quo to be an acceptable part of your lifestyle.

In this section, starting with this chapter, I want to share some of the benefits that you can expect from exercise. I have always referred to exercise as the *fitness twin* to diet. When working in concert with each other, these twins can create both short- and long-term results just like the combat twins we read about earlier for your emotional well-being.

I think it is fair to say that most people do not like the thought of exercise—at least that is the feedback I have received from people I've come in contact with for many years. And if you, too, dread the thought of exercise, please stick around because there is so much in store for you if you just give it a try. I know it is very difficult to start a physically active lifestyle when you have been living a sedentary lifestyle. But with a change of mind and willingness to at least try, you will soon find out that getting off the couch will be the most difficult exercise you will have to do—the rest gets easier day by day. And when the thought of going to the gym becomes greater than the purpose for going there, re-read the Attitude section of this book and then remember the mantra: *Focus on the purpose not the task!* You are not alone when it comes to dealing with making yourself overcome negative thoughts—we all deal with that, and we always will. It is a part of life. We all need to exercise to enhance the quality of our lives.

> With a change of mind and willingness to at least try, you will soon find out that getting off the couch will be the most difficult exercise you will have do

With a change of mind and willingness to at least try, you will soon find out that getting off the couch will be the most difficult exercise you will have do—the rest gets easier day by day.

Physiological Benefits

Exercising your body is not about hard work, but rather about being smarter by applying compatible exercises that work best for your body genetics. Whether your interests are to feel better, improve your illness profile, lose weight, maintain weight, redesign your physique, or just burn off the stress of the day, exercise will be your reliable companion for life. It will never fail you. Let's see what your benefits package has to offer you:

▸ Cardiovascular system—Heart muscle function is improved by exercise. A conditioned heart is capable of handling physical stress more efficiently and recovers more quickly (improved resting heart rate). A strong heart is more likely to rebound after a heart attack.

▸ Circulatory system—Exercise increases the flow of blood throughout the body, enhances energy, and promotes stamina. It positively effects sexual health, mental health, and removes toxins from your body. It also delivers and nourishes every living cell in your body with oxygen, vitamins, minerals, and other nutrients. (One reason dietary supplements and eating foods for your blood type are so important.)

▶ Pulmonary system—Exercise increases lung capacity, enhances stamina, and endurance. Exercise creates more energy, not less! Walking stairs, going bowling, and playing various sports rids the body of toxins and keeps the lungs healthy.

▶ Digestive system—This system is improved enormously through exercise, which helps remove dangerous toxicity build up in the colon. It normalizes bowel movement and greatly enhances regularity and proper bowel function. Exercise also helps with eliminating water retention.

▶ Detoxification system—A natural cleansing occurs as exercise promotes perspiration, which causes your body to rid itself of toxins, water retention, salts, and cellular debris (all toxins).

▶ Lymphatic system—Exercise detoxifies the lymphatic system as well as flushing other vital organs.

▶ Exercise helps stabilize the blood sugar level, which is good for diabetics, people with insulin problems, and hypoglycemia. It allows constant energy flow throughout the day and enhances weight loss.

▶ Exercise promotes healthier skin and skin tone by increasing blood flow closer to the surface skin.

▸ Exercise slows down the aging process. Improves mental alertness and prevents or slows down the onset of mental illnesses that are common today, like Alzheimer's and dementia.

▸ Exercise strengthens muscles, ligaments, and cartilage; improves joint mobility and flexibility; and promotes bone density, which prevents the onset of osteoporosis.

▸ Exercise raises your HDL (good cholesterol) and helps reduce your LDL (bad cholesterol). HDL helps remove plaque in the arteries LDL (bad cholesterol). The net result is a better HDL/cholesterol ratio and lower risk of heart disease, diabetes, stroke, and a host of other potential medical ailments.

Blood Pressure

Exercise contributes to lowering blood pressure. As blood and oxygen flow is increased from exercise, the blood vessels dilate to accommodate the body's demands. HDL (good cholesterol) goes up, cleansing or vacuuming the blood vessels whereby buildup of plaque or saturated fat is carried away. In return, this allows the heart to pump blood through the arteries more efficiently and with less resistance which contributes to lowering your blood pressure reading.

Metabolism

Metabolic activity is everything when it comes to losing weight and exercise boosts your metabolism. Exercise improves your BMR (basal metabolic rate), your body's ability to burn calories while resting by developing lean muscle mass. Exercise is absolutely imperative for weight loss because it improves your body composition (lean weight vs. body fat) requiring more calories to burn twenty-four hours a day. As you develop a positive body composition, an increase in muscle tissue, and reduction in body fat percentage, your body becomes the natural calorie burner it was designed to be. This removes all the unnecessary work most people endure when attempting to lose weight. When the body mechanics for losing weight are properly operating, the results are weight loss and weight maintenance. Instead of dieting and exercising to lose weight, really all you have to do is to get the parts operating properly. The rest is natural and easy—I know!

Your metabolism is stimulated during exercise, assisting in utilizing stored calories for energy. A revved metabolism through exercise promotes fat loss as opposed to a dead metabolism which stores fat! Afterwards, when you are through exercising your body continues to burn calories at an accelerated pace for some thirty to sixty minutes!

Your three-fold metabolic benefit package from exercise:

1. Your metabolism is revved during your workout or physical activity, which utilizes stored fat for the energy to perform the exercises.

2. There is an after-calorie burning effect for up to an hour or so after your workout is over, causing your body to continue to burn fat calories after you stop exercising.

3. By developing a positive body composition (increased lean muscle mass and less body fat) through exercise, your body burns calories more efficiently twenty-four hours per day, which means while you are sleeping, sitting at your desk, or lying on the couch your body is burning calories—not storing them!

Recap of your package: Exercise promotes weight loss, produces a positive body composition, builds muscle, strengthens the immune system, and improves the cardiovascular system, the digestive system, and circulatory system. It assists diabetic and hypoglycemic conditions by stabilizing blood sugar levels. It promotes more energy and stamina, lowers blood pressure and cholesterol, and helps reverse the effects of aging. What more could you want? Sounds like an impressive benefits package to me!

Real People, Real Results

Over the years I have received numbers of testimonials via e-mail, letters, and phone calls from people who have experienced both the health and cosmetic benefits that come from making food choices based on their blood type and exercise programs based on their body genetics. Results may vary per individual due to one's particular circumstances, current condition of health, exercise history, genetic individuality, illness profile, and attitude. Still, we all have a potential that can be reached.

You do not need to be a fitness guru or expert to reach your genetic potential. You won't need to spend every spare moment in the gym and you certainly do not have to diet to lose weight and keep it off. The information you have received in this book will lead you to maximizing your genetic potential to be all that you are capable of being.

You start off with high expectations of what you want to look like or feel like. Shortly afterwards the dark cloud of uncertainty may disrupt your vision as to whether you will actually reach your goals. Let me assure you that there is a light at the end of the tunnel and your goals are attainable…**if** you stay the course. Certainly the baseline or foundation to succeed won't be built on a generic module or model but rather on your genetic individuality. With your new **Never Go Back** attitude and emotional stability, you can reach your goal because you have the tools to make that come true. If you want to redesign your body, lose weight and keep it off, or improve your illness profile, learning more about yourself and knowing how to identify your genetic characteristics are the keys for lifelong success.

Reading what others have to say about their results and experiences always helps to motivate and give hope to the one who is ready to venture out on their journey. Certainly seeing the success that others have experienced is extremely inspiring.

To keep you pumped up and encouraged before you start out on the journey of taking your body, mind, and spirit to another level, I chose to list several individuals with whom I have had the privilege to share my insights and expertise over the years. Their experiences and success are representative of the *inspiration in transition* role models they truly have become. And they are willing to share their experiences with you.

As you read the testimonials and look at the "before and after" photos, keep in mind that at some point in their lives they wanted to improve their health, quality of life, and the way they looked…just like you. The difference is that they went forward and did something about it. Their experience and success was not an accident, but is the fruit of their labor. Their reward wasn't a slice of chocolate cake, but the results they experienced—and so will yours. Like them, you can expect maximum results as you factor your genetic individuality into making food selections and exercise programs.

Testimonials

No More GERD

> *My husband and I have taken all the information from your books very seriously and have been using the food plan for our blood type for only a couple weeks. I stopped craving sweet simple carbohydrates and my husband no longer has GERD or sinus problems. We are convinced that our blood types are crucial to what we eat.*
>
> —PJ from CA

No More Respiratory, No More Asthma Medication

I am type O; Apple body type and am 63 years old. I switched to eating for my blood type 100%. I have cut back on my thyroid medication and am off my asthma and respiratory medications. I no longer have hypoglycemia. I have increased my exercise regime for the Apple body type and have lost four inches around the waist.
—C, Department of Veterans Affairs

No More Discomfort

*In 1981 I was diagnosed with cancer, and am now completely healed and enjoying good health. Going through this experience made me appreciate my health and quality of life. When I found out my blood type I realized that I was eating incorrectly for my type and my body was reacting to it. In six months after following your book (Bloodtypes, Bodytypes and YOU) my life has changed for the better. I determined in my heart that I would eat beneficial foods and avoid the Avoid foods, and within 3 days I began to experience the results. I had previously experienced a lot of stomach disorders and was hospitalized on several occasions and discharged because the doctors couldn't determine the cause. Now all the symptoms are gone and my energy is great. In addition to feeling good and having higher energy, I have lost 2 dress sizes. **I haven't given up anything except discomfort***
—L. from Florida

Mother and Daughter Lose 218 Pounds in One Year!

I tried other diets but they did not work. But this was so easy to do. It was not hard at all. When I started, I set a goal to lose weight and be healthier by my 50ᵗʰ birthday (August 2004). Heart trouble and high blood pressure run in my family. My mother was having health problems so I started her eating for her blood type also. After one year I have lost 118 pounds and my mother has lost 100 pounds. We both have more energy and are in better health. My mother is no longer on medications and her doctor said, "Whatever you are doing, keep doing it." Both of us follow your 80/20 rule for eating and exercising for our body types. It has been a blessing and is so much better than our old lifestyle.

—Gail and Jean W., Virginia

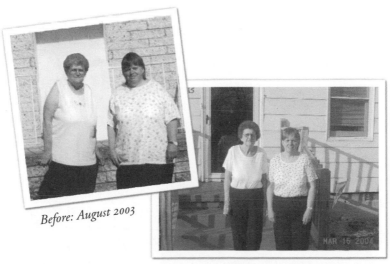

Before: August 2003

After: August 2004

Simple and Easy

I was so skeptical at first about this genetic thing with food and exercise but followed the food plans from your book. It has changed my life!!! The things on the Avoid list have always been a problem for me: corn, orange juice, vinegar, peanuts, Brussels sprouts, dairy foods, etc. The things I didn't realize were bad for me were wheat, potatoes and pasta, which I was eating a lot of because I thought they were healthy foods. I have suffered with allergies, thyroid disease, constipation, bloating, gas, and colitis.

I have been on the exercise program for 5 weeks and I cannot believe the change. I lost 2 inches in my waist the first 4 weeks! I have not eaten anything on my Avoid list and for the first 4 weeks I tried to eat only beneficial foods. I felt so good, I just couldn't make myself not continue. Thank you for making this so simple and easy and for giving me the tools to live a healthy life!

—B, Texas

Let the Results Speak for Themselves

When I saw Joe Christiano on a television program about three years ago I decided to buy his book (Bloodtypes, Bodytypes and YOU).

I did the typical, "Look to see what foods I should avoid based on my blood type" scan of the book. I didn't like everything I saw but went ahead and read the book and at least gave it a try. Instead of focusing on the "avoid" foods for being a blood type A, I simply began to switch to more of the beneficial and neutral foods. It was refreshing to try some new foods that I liked. Already in good health, I noticed my energy level increase more than anything. I didn't seem to have the crashing feeling after a meal at all now. My metabolism increased as I noticed more definition in my body. I eat probably 80 - 90% according to my blood type and don't feel like I'm depriving myself. I also began to adjust my exercises a little to include those suitable for my body type and renewed my interest in competing in a body building contest.

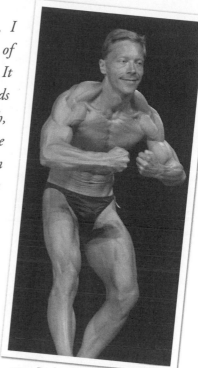

2005 Body Building Champion

So at age 42, I entered the 2005 Potomac Cup Drug Free competition. By the grace of God, the support of my wife and daughter, and the advice, expertise and encouragement of Dr. Joe, I won the lightweight novice division, the 40 and over pose-down, and finished third in the Master's 35 division.

I have a passion to see people live up to their full God-given potential in every area: spirit, soul, and body.

—Pastor Rocky, Virginia

Blood Type O

I just wanted to express my thanks to you for putting this program on the market. My husband (blood type B) and I started this one month ago. We have experienced great results. My husband has lost 16.5 inches over his total body, 7% body fat, and 5 pounds. I have lost 28 inches over my total body, 10.25% body fat, and 10 pounds. This is all in just the first month. Needless to say, we are continuing with the program and have also shared it with my parents, and also my brother and his wife, as well as several friends. Again, thank you for the program.

—B, Tennessee

New shape

I purchased your exercise tape in June of 2001, and have continued to follow the exercise for the "Pear Shape." I have dropped from a size 18 to a 12-14, and have lost about 36 pounds. This is the first time I have experienced a vast difference in the shape of my lower body. Years ago I walked 3 miles a day at a fast pace, 5-6 days a week, for 2-3 years, and did not see the results that I have experienced now. A friend told me that I had a "straight up and down" shape now. Thank you.

—H. B.

Blood Type O

I have been on your weight management program since February 2002. I lost 18 pounds and feel great. I really never looked overweight but I am 5'4" and weighed 150 pounds and now I weigh 132 and I have lost inches. I went from a size 12 to an 8. I am 46 and look 36. I have tried it all and let me tell you this program is a way of life for me! Thank you for making losing weight a no-brainer.

—K

No Stomach Discomfort

I had a lot of digestive problems and some pain in my stomach, which I believe was an ulcer(for years). Since I started eating more food for my blood type (A), I am doing much better and NO stomach discomfort! Thank you so much

—O M, Dallas, Texas

Husband and Wife—It's a Lifestyle Now!

We weren't looking for another diet and exercise program. We've done them all! What we were looking for was a baby. Rod and I have struggled with infertility since 1998 when I was diagnosed with a tumor on my pituitary gland. It wreaked havoc on my hormonal system and caused my progesterone level to be quite low. Conception was very difficult. It also caused weight gain, which added to my depression. Then in August of 1999 my mother passed away from cancer of the brain. My anxiety, stress and weight were at an all-time high.

Rod and I were both increasingly disgusted with our bodies because of poor eating habits and little or no physical activity. We had low energy and little willpower to resist the foods that were causing our "growing" problem. It seemed overwhelming at times.

When we were introduced to the concept of eating according to our blood type, we were both a bit skeptical. We made the mistake of looking first at the Avoid lists and began to protest. But after about a week of eating mostly beneficial and some neutral foods for my blood type, I stopped craving the nachos I had to have! Our energy levels increased incredibly, and combined with the exercises Dr. Joe showed us, we had amazing results.

In twelve weeks we lost fat and inches, gained muscle and improved our health. Rod lost forty-two pounds of fat and normalized his cholesterol (which was high prior to this) and his blood pressure. I lost thirty pounds of fat, gained five pounds of muscle, went down three dress sizes and lost forty-seven total inches of body size. We like having the three-month goal as a motivation, and when we finish three months, we just start three more. I needed hope again. And I found it by changing my lifestyle. It really is a lifestyle for us now.

—Stacy and Rod

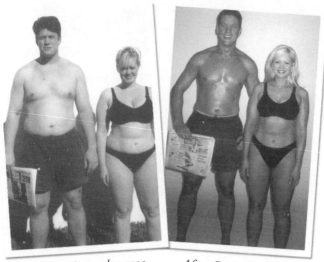

Before: September 1999   *After: December 1999*

In just twelve weeks I went from 23 percent body fat to under 10 percent, lost forty-two pounds of fat and went from a tight size forty pants to a very comfortable thirty-six. I am six foot four inches tall and weigh 225 pounds, so a thirty-six is pretty good!

All the fat loss was great, awesome and all of that, but the real story is our energy levels and our health. Not only did our energy levels stabilize but they went through the roof. I am a full-time youth pastor, a part-time Terminator at University Studios in Florida and a full-time husband. My lifestyle demands a lot from me. My wife is a full-time singer/entertainer and a wonderful wife, so hers is equally demanding. Let's just say that energy is not a problem anymore!

We really feel good. We look better, so we feel better about ourselves. All areas of our lives have improved. We are both more confident and less inhibited to try new things. Now that we have done this whole body redesign, we have found that if we can discipline ourselves in one area of our lives, we can do it in any area. Not only are our bodies in better shape—our lives are in better shape. We can do anything we put our minds to! We are so proud of each other, and we have a greater respect for each other. Every part of our relationship has improved. We are so glad we met Dr. Joe, he has been a very big help to us!

—Rod

Others noticed something different

One year ago I was extremely overweight and had no energy. My lifestyle consisted of consuming eight to twelve cans of Diet Pepsi a day and eating a lot of food packed with fat, sugars and no nutrients.

I began following Dr. Joe's program of eating according to my blood type and exercising according to my body type on a regular basis. I noticed immediate results. Within three weeks, I had blood work done, and my cholesterol had dropped over sixty points. When I went to the doctor's office for the lab results, she burst into the room saying, "I am thrilled at the results of your blood work. Whatever you are doing, keep it up."

Prior to embracing this lifestyle, I had my thyroid removed. My doctor has consistently lowered my medication since I began the program because my body is more in line with the way it should be. Another benefit was the immediate increased energy I felt. I no longer dreaded getting out of bed and dragging myself through the day. The exercise became a part of my daily routine, and very soon I felt something was missing on the days I could not exercise.

I do not have a scale, and really don't know how much weight I've lost; however, I have lost six dress sizes. Even during Thanksgiving and Christmas holidays I continued to lose sizes. We went to more Christmas parties than we had ever attended, and I ate a lot of food. But I just ate food appropriate for blood type O as much as possible.

Since I have lost so many sizes it is not difficult for others to notice that something is different. I enjoy sharing with them the secrets to my success—eating and exercising according to my type.

—Debbie

Keeping if off for 8 years!

It is amazing how one person can change your life forever, give you a positive outlook and help you achieve your goals. I never had a weight problem as a child. That is, until I became a teenager. My hormones kicked in and took my body through many changes of which forty to fifty pounds was one of them. I wore baggy clothes so that people wouldn't notice. When people looked at me, I thought they were looking at my weight—not at me as a person. Because of that I lost a lot of self-confidence.

Throughout high school and college I was very active, playing softball, cheerleading and dancing, but something was still missing. I tried so many different diet plans, pills and programs, but nothing helped—it only got worse. I would lose a little weight and then put it right back on. I couldn't find a program that catered to my needs, body and schedule. I felt overwhelmed and lost.

I had a lot of friends and enjoyed being with people, but deep down inside, I realized I wasn't happy with myself. I knew that one of the most important parts of life was to love me for who I was.

I had many goals in life, and one of them was to compete in the Miss New York USA Pageant. I've been involved in pageants since I was thirteen, but I would not compete if there was a swimsuit competition. I am very goal-oriented, but how could I compete in the pageant when I was overweight?

I had seen Dr. Joe Christiano and read his articles in several editions of a pageant magazine, and the work he had done with pageant contestants. The pictures accompanying the articles were amazing. With some of the women, the transition from before to after was unbelievable. I thought if I was going to achieve my goals, a good place to start would be by giving Joe a call. That call- changed my life.

As a health and fitness life coach, I talked extensively with Joe over the phone, and within a few weeks, I was on a regular workout schedule and diet program—not a diet—it was more like an eating regimen.

Joe and I talked at least once a week for the first month, and then once or twice a month thereafter. At any given time, though, if I felt discouraged or needed encouragement, he was always there to help. He was very encouraging, supportive and motivating. Whenever I needed him, he was always there—even when I wanted to quit.

I saw results in the first month and within months after dropping thirty pounds and seventeen and a half inches I was walking down the runway at the Miss New York USA Pageant—my self-esteem and confidence just in taking that walk were amazing.

I was at a standstill; I wasn't losing any more, and I had reached a plateau. That's when he introduced me to eating according to my blood type a program genetically designed to target my specific blood type. My eating habits changed once again. Foods that before I thought were good for me now actually had a negative effect on my body. This meant that they were not being properly digested.

At the same time, Dr. Joe tweaked my workout program to target specific areas of my body that needed to be redesigned. What a difference it made. I was losing body fat, not muscle fat. My muscles were more defined and lean. I felt great.

When I wanted to give up, Dr. Joe wouldn't let me. He lent himself to me as a mentor, friend, and personal fitness coach. He never let me become disillusioned with myself. There were pep talks to bolster my self-image and positive encouragement to help me build my self-confidence and continue with my determination to reach my goals. He possessed the very important skill of being a great listener.

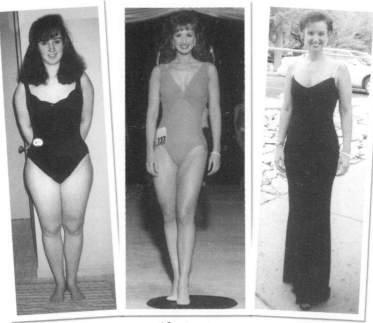

Before: 1998   *After: 1999*   *Present: 2006*

My attitude and personality changed dramatically. I learned proper eating habits and ways to work out and challenge my body based on my genetic makeup.

Today, eight years later at 33 years old, I still have maintained my weight at 138 pounds. I continue with the techniques I've learned from Dr. Joe and model my life around those techniques. I don't panic if I gain a few pounds for one reason or another because I have a solid foundation of knowledge and expertise to support me. I exercise 4-5 times a week, including cardio, weights and various machines. This is very important to me to maintain my weight but also it's a great stress reliever.

Thank you again for all your support and encouragement. You have truly made a difference in my life.
—Lynn, lwesley@rnews.com

The names may have been changed only to protect the privacy of those who so willingly submitted their experiences. Some testimonials have been edited to accommodate space.

— Renewing Your Mind —

() There is no question that exercising can be a tough decision to commit to especially if you are living a sedentary lifestyle. Does the thought of exercise overwhelm your mind to the point that you find it hard to commit to? Yes, or no? If your answer is yes, then do what everyone who makes exercise a part of their lifestyle—look at the benefit package! See if you can identify with the Real People, Real Results above for inspiration and motivation. The goal is not to be a 90-day makeover wonder, but to cross the finish line a winner!

() It may be hard for you to grasp this concept if you have not yet made exercise a part of your lifestyle but it is almost equally mental as it is physical. Do you have certain goals or dreams of what you would like to look like? Yes, or no? If you do not then let me suggest that you review the Attitude section to help you establish a reason and motivation to go for it. As a professional and veteran I have to refresh my attitude and refocus my sights when it comes to exercising. Remember: *Focus on the purpose not the task*! That mantra is painted on the wall of my home gym because I too, need to be reminded of my purpose(s) while going through the tasks.

() Goals need to be set in increments. Yes, it would be nice to wave a wand and immediately attain your goals, but that is not a reality. Reaching your genetic potential is a reality. Establishing short-term goals is not only fulfilling and rewarding, but helps sets a precedent for making lifelong goals a reality. Would you like to achieve your very own '"before and after" photo? If so, take a closer look at the "before" and "after" photos of the people in this chapter for motivation and inspiration. They did it. I did it and you will do it, too! But remember: your "before" photo is your reminder of where you once were—a place of dreams and hopes. Your "after" photo is your reminder that you can do what you set your mind to do and are living out your dreams and hopes.

Exercise: You don't have time not to.

—Unknown

Chapter

14

Things to Know Before You Exercise

I HAVE SEEN IT OVER AND OVER. WHENEVER A PERSON IS READY TO make a change in their lifestyle—whether it is to lose weight, be more physically fit, or improve their overall health—there is a tendency to jump in head over heels. Their intention was good but what they needed was to be better prepared. Their zeal got ahead of their knowledge and consequently their lifelong dream never became a reality. **I don't want this to happen to you.**

Be "In the Know"

There is no generic or one-size-fits-all approach to diet or exercise. I believe most well-intended individuals have suffered through diet and exercise by not realizing the major role their genetic individuality plays. It is the missing link that must be factored not only into your diet but also into your exercise plan for the most success. You are not the same as the next person (even a family member), so you will not respond the same way as they do, whether from diet and nutrition or from physical exercise. If you maintain that old school of thought then you may do well, but most likely you will not attain your personal goal of redesigning your body and maintaining it for life.

> You are not the same as the next person, so you will not respond the same way as they do.

The next chapter will show how your genetics play such an important role in redesigning your body with accuracy and individuality. But before we study the uniqueness of your genetic characteristics, there are some basics that need to be addressed regardless of your goals or your genetics.

Let's look at some *basic generic principles* that will help broaden your scope of knowledge and preparedness before you travel down the road that leads to a successful body redesigning journey.

Progressive Fitness Principles

Principle # 1: *Exercise a minimum of three times weekly.* If you exercise fewer than three days per week, you might find it difficult to get fit and lose body fat. On the other hand, you should start out slowly but progressively, allowing only what your fitness condition dictates. Too much too fast will cause potential injury and burnout, and will lead to frustration and eventual dropout.

Principle # 2: ***Exercise for a minimum of fifteen minutes.***
Recent research has shown that as few as twelve minutes of
exercise per session can produce cardiovascular improvement
(stamina but not much fat reduction). To assure more fat reduction, try aerobic training, which is low in intensity and long in
duration. Then you will be able to exercise longer.

Principle #3: ***Warm up and cool down.*** Ideally, a 10-15 minute
warm up of walking or cycling prepares the heart, lungs, and
muscles for a vigorous workout. It raises your core body tempera-
ture, which puts your body into a fat-burning mode. After your
workout is over, it is a good idea to slow down the pace and cruise
for about ten minutes or so. Stretching is a perfect way to cool
down. This gives your internal machinery time to recover at an
easy pace. Having a cool down period assists in eliminating much
of the lactic acid buildup in the muscle tissue incurred during the
main exercise time.

Principle #4: ***Drink water to stay hydrated.*** Start out with an
eight to ten ounce glass of water, about twenty minutes before
each workout session. Then continue to drink water during the
workout. It is important to stay hydrated. Immediately after your
exercise session, make sure you drink more water. Don't wait
until you get thirsty to hydrate. Instead, drink water throughout
the activity.

Pay close attention to the environment around you. If you are
exercising outdoors and it's hot and humid, you might be wise to

go indoors or pass on the workout completely unless your body is used to the heat. Otherwise, your body will have a difficult time cooling down in those conditions. Make sure you drink more than normal throughout those days. In fact increase your daily water consumption to half of your body weight (converted into ounces). (See Appendix A for more information about alkaline water—my personal choice for drinking water.)

Principle # 5: ***Practice safety during exercise.*** Monitor your heart rate throughout your workout sessions and stay within your ideal range. Remember to breathe and not hold your breath during an exercise movement. Sometimes people unconsciously hold their breath while exercising. This may cause elevated blood pressure, and you won't last long without a constant flow of oxygen. Concentrate on exercise technique and form. This will minimize the potential of injury and will produce the best results.

Principle # 6: ***Do a variety of exercises.*** Follow a baseline of exercises at least three times per week, but mix it up on the other days. Add recreational activities like biking or hiking. Play some tennis or volleyball. Keep it interesting by varying your activities. Keep moving!

Principle # 7: ***Include family and friends.*** The nice thing about exercising is that it can be social. Some prefer to go it alone, but it is fun to share this positive experience with like-minded people. For couples, evening walks become a means for having quality time after work hours. Walks during lunch breaks make for a great way to connect with fellow employees and burn those calories.

Parents must get involved in their children's lives and doing physical activities with them is one great way. Get the kids away from the TV, game boys, and the video games. Take them outside and play tennis or volleyball, take walks, throw the football around, or exercise together. Get creative so all the things you do are enjoyable for boys or girls. Their health is in your hands.

Your program should have the simplicity and flexibility to be conducted in the privacy of your home or at a health club, whichever you prefer. It need not require complicated or expensive equipment. Your program should also be a time saver. Most people do not have a lot of time to spare, so keep it short but effective. Then you will be able to stay motivated for the long haul. (See Appendix B *Fork in the Road*.)

Three Components of an Exercise Program

It is obviously impossible for me to design a personal exercise program for everyone who reads this book. However, I can give you an idea of what your body requires and what an exercise program should provide you.

All exercise programs should consist of the following three components:

(1) **Cardiovascular Conditioning**—enhances your stamina and endurance by improving your VO2 uptake, or your ability to take

in oxygen. As your cardio-respiratory system (heart and lungs and circulatory system) improve so does your ability to recover from physical exertion. Exercises such as walking, jogging, jumping rope, circuit training, or exercise equipment such as stationary bikes, treadmills, and/or elliptical machines are all cardiovascular-specific activities for improving your cardiovascular condition. Cardiovascular conditioning occurs when you remain active at a heart rate of sixty to seventy percent of your maximum heart rate.

The benefits of cardiovascular conditioning include strengthening the heart and lungs, improving circulation, reducing cholesterol levels and body fat percentage, and improving your ability to recover from physical exertion. When doing moderate intensity exercise such as cardiovascular conditioning, fat is the primary energy source used by the body for fuel—making this a good fat-burning activity.

(2) **Strength or Resistance Training**—improves your muscle size, shape, and strength through continual resistance. Exercises that enhance a muscle's ability to exert force against resistance produce strength. Isometric exercises, negative resistance training, gravitational exercises, and manual resistance exercises are good examples of strength training. Examples of equipment that can be used for resistance training are the multi-station exercise machines, conventional machines using cables and pulleys with weight stacks, plate-loaded equipment, and handy free weights such as barbells or dumbbells—all are tools of the trade for strength training.

Strength training shapes and tones muscles and makes them stronger. Strength training will help elevate your good cholesterol (HDL) levels, which in turn contributes to lowering the bad cholesterol (LDL). Strength training stimulates your metabolic rate for burning fat calories. Strength training also aids in the prevention of injury by promoting proper balance among the various muscle groups. Your body composition improves due to strength training by increasing the lean muscle tissue and lowering the body fat percent.

(3) **Flexibility Training**—This type of training enhances and promotes the ability to move a joint through the full range of motion (ROM) without discomfort. Full range of motion for every joint is a must for proper joint action. Physical inactivity promotes poor range of motion in the joints, joint stiffness, and pain. Adding flexibility training or stretching to your daily routine is highly recommended. With all of the yoga classes available now, you might want to try one of those for improving your flexibility.

(3a) **Stretching**—Static stretching is a form of stretching that gently promotes elongation and flexibility of muscle and soft tissue. This form of stretching is gentle and relaxing and is the opposite of ballistic stretching that calls for a bouncing motion. Again, this is where some yoga can be effective.

When stretching a muscle, stretch it until it becomes comfortably tight but not painfully uncomfortable. Do not jerk the limbs you are stretching, but simply apply a constant, gentle stretch. Be careful not to stretch beyond that comfort point or you will not be able to relax the muscle and not benefit from the stretching exercise.

The benefits from stretching or flexibility training are a decrease in muscle and joint injury and soreness, lengthening of muscle and connective tissue, and lubricating the dry joint area. Stretching will reduce stress and anxiety while teaching you how to relax.

Note: I recommend that you warm up the muscles first, then stretch them out. For example, the next time you decide to jog or power walk, it would be wise to walk gently for about ten minutes. Warm up those calf muscles by pumping blood into them and lubricate those joints by inducing synovial fluid. Then, after the short warm-up or pre-workout session, take time to stretch the muscles involved in your workout for that session.

Properly stretched muscles will perform at their optimum. Golfing, bowling, tennis, hiking, dancing, chasing the kids around—everything will become easier when your muscles are flexible.

Exercise and Functional Age

I realize nobody wants to talk about or even think about the fact that they are getting older. When you watch TV or go to the movies you see ultra-thin Hollywood personalities. They are thin, shapely, and young. They share their workout programs, special diets and all the extra things they do to stay in fantastic shape in the magazines—but they are young. They should be shapely.

What about the rest of us who are older than that younger generation and are dealing with our age, the aging process, and the way our bodies act and react lately? There is nothing you can do about the clock on the wall or your chronological age. You are as old as you are, but you can do something about your physical fitness condition at your age. The older you get, the more important it becomes for you to exercise.

Many of us think the aging process doesn't begin until we reach our parents' age but the truth is that the aging process actually begins immediately after birth. But for this book, let's just suppose that it begins in the twenties. Often we are unaware of the aging process until we hit our forties, which is when many of the anti-aging hormones drop off significantly.

As we age, our bodies become more fragile because our activity levels decrease. We sit more and move less. Our bones are deteriorating through demineralization. This sedentary lifestyle with its lack of physical activity contributes to the dysfunction and ill-health of the joints—knees, ankles, hips, shoulders, elbows, and spine. Even day-to-day tasks can become a burden. This condition is compounded by a loss of muscle tissue/mass (or muscle atrophy) because of lack of physical activity. Physical inactivity is the nemesis to a successful weight loss / management lifestyle. On top of that, it messes with our mental attitude and we all know the importance of maintaining the right attitude—don't we?

If that isn't enough, there are other factors such our genetic individuality/heredity, gender, physical injuries, and overall lifestyle practices that need to be considered. Finally, throw in a litany of premature chronic diseases and you have just lowered your *functional age*. *Functional age* is your ability to physically function at a younger age than your actual chronological age. Functional age is based on your physical fitness. If you are actively involved in regular exercise, you will reduce your functional age. On the contrary, by living a sedentary lifestyle you will raise your functional age.

For example, if you are a forty-five-year-old who does not exercise and lacks fitness, I guarantee you probably feel and move like a sixty-year-old person instead of the forty-five-year-old person you are. On the other hand, if you are a sixty-year-old who exercises regularly and are in good shape, you may very well function as a thirty-year-old. Keep in mind that your functional age is determined by other factors such as genetics, environmental adaptations, etc., but exercise plays a huge role.

What's the big deal about getting older anyway? It's not what age you are, but what you do with what you have! So, do something about it. Exercise regularly!

To help you better prepare yourself before you exercise, read through some of the following things to consider as you take the road that leads you to becoming healthier and more physically fit as you mature.

▶ See a doctor before beginning your exercise program, especially if you are over thirty-five and have been inactive for several years. It's good to have a birds-eye view of what is going on inside and the assurance of a health care professional.

▶ Factor in your age before jumping into any exercise program. I have worked with many young mid-thirty-year old men and women who nearly bought the farm because they forgot they weren't spring chickens anymore! Consider your age, your current activity level, and overall fitness level beforehand.

▶ How long has it been since you trained with free weights or exercise equipment on a regular basis? Are you making a comeback, or are you a beginner? Don't expect to reach your goals in one workout. Regardless of your exercise background, your long-term success must begin **one** step at a time.

▶ Are you interested in getting in shape to assist your athletic ability and performance? If so, then your training program must be designed for sports or sports specific.

▶ Are you a female and have specific goals like getting into a smaller dress size or losing a certain amount of weight so you can wear those clothes that are still hanging in your closet since you gained weight? Then your exercise protocol must be designed to accommodate and assist in body fat reduction.

▸ Are you lacking energy, strength or balance in your physique? Again, these areas of concern and interest must be factored into your exercise strategy before you start. Should the program place the emphasis on cardiovascular conditioning or on strength training and body redesigning? Find the answer for your body type.

▸ What are your body genetic limitations? Do you know how to troubleshoot your genetic problem areas? Your program must be tailored to your body genetic specifics or you will be spinning your wheels and your results will be very, very slow.

▸ Have fun with exercise. Your regular program should be designed to meet your specific goals, but be sure to stay physically active in addition to your program.

▸ Be sure to throw in some physical activities outside the gym, such as tennis, volleyball, golf, or any other sport or activity that you enjoy and will keep the blood flowing.

Staying physically active is key to higher energy, less body fat, better appearance, less illness, longevity, and a host of other benefits. Take the time to apply this information to your lifestyle.

In the next chapter you will see that I have gone from using generic exercise information to being more accurate and specific about redesigning your body by factoring in your genetic individuality. Through learning how to identify with your unique body genetics and the role they play in the outcome of your efforts, you will see how this approach refutes the one-fits-all approach.

(See Appendix B, *Fork in the Road* life-coaching series on attitude, diet, and exercise for a more in-depth coaching experience on the above.)

— Renewing Your Mind —

() Are you a beginner when it comes to exercise? Yes, or no? If yes, then the first step you took had to be mental or attitude. You had to decide to go for it. Now, instead of diving in head first, be smart and acquaint yourself with the practical tips and suggestions from this chapter. As a beginner you want to remember to take it **one day at a time**. Your body has to adjust to the physical changes and so does your mind. Keep in mind that you should progress according to your current condition including physical limitations, time restraints, etc. Again, the more you know about what you are about to venture into the better the outcome. This is truly an investment of your time, energy, and money!

() The clock is ticking on the wall and you and I can do nothing to stop it. But we can do something about the manner in which we age. As you get older wouldn't you like to age gracefully and with as much youthfulness and vigor as you can have? I will assume your answer is yes! Combining exercise and a healthy lifestyle is the ticket to make that dream come true. As you age chronologically—getting older—you can actually function…younger. If you take a moment and observe our older people in their seventies and eighties, you can easily see that they are limited to what they can do just by their inability to move around. Canes and walkers seem to be the apparatus of choice for them. But my contention is if they would simply exercise regularly (even at their age) their muscles, ligaments, and tendons would be much stronger and everyday tasks would be easier and less painful. I know you may not be there yet, but someday you will be. Now is the time to make exercise a daily part of your lifestyle. As you grow older, live younger!

Our bodies are our gardens to which our wills are gardeners.

—William Shakespeare

Chapter

15

Discover the Real You

THIS CHAPTER CONTAINS SOME SPECIFIC THINGS ABOUT yourself that you may not be aware of when it comes to your body, its genetic design, and how to go about redesigning it. Exercising your body certainly delivers many benefits. But I think you will agree that one of the benefits most appealing to everyone is having a new shape or new body. I refer to it as body redesigning.

There's More to You Than You May Know!

Body redesigning does not come by accident, but rather from a well-planned out methodology of exercise know-how that is compatible to one's body genetics. I know because I have been redesigning bodies for years and years (See *Real People, Real Results*.)

Body redesigning is the most likely motive for going to the gym over any other. But, a redesigned body takes more than just exercising or working hard. The success that I have experienced both in my own life and those I have coached and/or trained comes from my ability to identify the person's body genetics—including body types, limitations, and problem areas. Once those areas are identified, the rest will follow suit.

> The answer to successfully redesigning your body will come from factoring in your genetic individuality along with a concerted effort to choose foods that are compatible to your specific blood type

Performing exercises that are compatible to your individual body genetics combined with the food selection for your blood type becomes the winning combination. It makes your approach to redesigning your body the most accurate for you. Of course there are other considerations such as physical limitations, schedules, history of exercise involvement, age, gender, etc., that need to be addressed. Nevertheless, the answer to successfully redesigning your body will come from factoring in your genetic individuality along with a concerted effort to choose foods that are compatible to your specific blood type.

Successfully redesigning your body is similar to going on a journey. Before you jump into the car, you should determine the direction you will take. You get a map to see how many miles you will be traveling, determine your travel time, and determine how much gas it will require. Will you be driving through the night or staying in a hotel, motel, or camp along the way? The point is that in order to have a successful journey you must be prepared so the trip is successful. The road to body redesigning is no different. It starts with knowing your unique body genetics (i.e, body type, metabolic type, blood type) plus any physical limitations that are associated with them. Once you have accomplished that phase the next step is to know which exercise protocol is best suited for your body genetics. Once you know what you have to work with, the rest of the journey will be a pleasant and rewarding experience.

Before you set out to reach your goals let me help you first prepare by looking at the different body types and see if you can identify yours. This information will give you the insights to better understanding what you need to do to redesign your unique body type. Review the Trouble Shooting Charts at the end of the chapter for each body type. As you identify with your body type you will understand why your body genetics are unique from the next.

Body Types

I have worked with many bodies from all walks of life and nearly all of them required anything from fine-tuning, a minor overhaul, or up to a major overhaul. Over the past thirty-five years I have helped pre-teens, grannies, and everyone in between to redesign their bodies. Yes, there are a very few blessed individuals who have the seemingly perfect symmetry and body balance and have done nothing to earn it. These are the ones who have bloomed from the womb and are exempt from spending much time and effort in trying to redesign their bodies. But for the majority of us, it is a different story.

How is it that someone you know (and we all know a person like this) can eat anything he or she desires and never puts on a pound? Or the total opposite people like me—all we have to do to make our waistlines grow is look at food? Do they know something we don't? Better yet, do they have something we don't?

It may seem to be a mystery, but as we investigate it further you will see how it makes sense that the answer is in a person's genes, or genetic makeup. Understanding your specific genetic characteristics and the role they play in your body type and shape will determine the outcome of your fitness efforts. As you apply the knowledge you are about to read, not only you will be less likely to get discouraged and give up, but you will feel more confident to push through all the obstacles. You will end up owning one of your own personally redesigned "after" photos.

Being able to redesign your body in a shorter time starts with knowing certain things about your body. Since seventy-five percent of your body genetics come straight from your parents' genes and not from what you have contributed, it is what you do with what you got that matters most! The key to reaching your genetic potential is to know your genetic individuality.

Genetic Individuality

For the most part, social and cultural influences determine what kind of "body look" is in vogue. It doesn't have much to do with biology and could very well be outdated or out of fashion in a couple of years. Striving to redesign your body to fit a look that contradicts your body type becomes a frustrating experience. Instead, aim to make the body you have as balanced, healthy, and as fit as possible.

Your body's genetic characteristics are what they are in spite of your level of motivation and effort to redesign your body. Generally most women want to attain the classic hourglass figure and men the V-shape, but your body type will dictate what you will need to do to accomplish that look.

Some body genetic characteristics are not so favorable. For example, consider that of a woman who has narrow clavicles (shoulder bones) and wide hips (pelvic bones). Because her upper body is narrower than her lower body, she is categorized as being a Pear-shaped body type. Her narrow shoulders and wide hipbones are predisposed genetic traits. These genetic characteristics are not favorable for naturally attaining that classic hourglass figure from generic exercises or an exercise program.

But the good news for this body type (or any body type) is there is hope because of the genetic potential that everyone possesses! By understanding her body type and her genetic individuality, she can still redesign her body to attain that hourglass figure. She can redesign her body and take her body to a level of shapeliness and symmetry that did not come with the original package. She just needs to know how to do so with the proper exercise for her body type.

The routine would be a combination of exercises for reducing the hips, thighs, and buttocks in combination with exercises for building the shoulders. Unless you know what you are doing, you will become a smaller Pear—not exactly what you set out to accomplish. Consequently there isn't much, if anything that can be done about redesigning the skeletal system or reducing the actual hipbones and elongating the clavicles. That is part of what you inherited from your parents that won't change. I suppose you can have some surgical procedure that can shave off some bone off your hips but that doesn't sound so practical. You may not outsmart your genes, but when you factor in your genetics and use specialized strategies that are compatible with them, you can enhance them to their fullest.

Body Types, Shapes, and Exercise

Your body type was in place when you were born. It was inherited from your parents just like the color of your eyes, your hair, and your height.

For years I have used the Pear, Apple, and Banana metaphors to help classify body shapes. Women and men share the genetic apple shape. The Apple shape is notorious for gaining weight around their upper torsos and midsections. They appear top heavy and have thin legs with no buttocks.

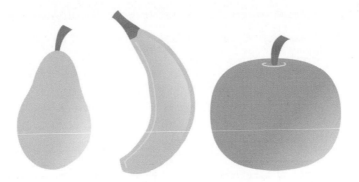

Women are generally pear-shaped, storing most of their excess body fat on their hips, thighs, and buttocks. They are often considered to be bottom heavy.

Then there is the Banana shape that is rather thin, with very few curves with a straight-lined physique. The Banana shape, like the Apple, is shared by both men and women.

The easiest way to determine your body shape is by answering the following question:

If I gain weight, where does most of it go?

- If you answer hips, thighs, and buttocks, you are a Pear.
- If you answer stomach, arms, and back, you are an Apple.
- If you answer both upper and lower, you are a Banana.

As you identify your genetic individuality, your journey toward redesigning your body is sure to be a successful trip. Exercises for each body shape are listed below. Look them over and see if you can identify with your unique body shape.

Note: Always consider your fitness condition—not the program—to dictate how much exercise to do. Start slowly and work up to the optimum exercises.

Apples

▸ *Aerobic sessions:* Try treadmill, stair climbing, or cycling. These sessions should be short in duration and high in intensity. Build up to thirty minutes at about sixty-five percent of your maximum heart rate. Adjust to your present physical fitness condition.

▸ *Cardiovascular Interval Training Sessions:* During a twenty- to twenty-five-minute workout, vary the intensity every few minutes. Exercise at sixty-five percent of your maximum heart rate for five minutes, then drop down to sixty percent again for the next five minutes. Continue varying your intensity for the whole workout.

▸ *Strength Training (Redesigning):* Concentrate on the upper torso, specifically on your shoulders, chest, and upper back. Keep the repetitions between fourteen and twenty-one, and perform three sets per exercise per body part. Start off at twenty to twenty-five minutes per workout. Since you are heavier on the top and taper down at the hips and thighs, you should concentrate on heavy lower body exercises. Try incorporating squats, leg presses, and calf raises. Do upper body exercises just for firming and toning the abs and pectorals.

Pears

▶ *Aerobic Sessions:* Try walking, cycling, or a treadmill. Your aerobic training sessions are nearly opposite to the apple's. The intensity level is low, which means you can train for a longer duration. Aerobic training done for a long period of time will help metabolize fat storage. The length of your aerobic session is an individual thing, but try for a minimum of thirty minutes. You can work up to forty-five minutes or sixty minutes if you are advanced and want to make significant improvements. Anything longer will not be as productive.

▶ *Cardiovascular Interval Training Sessions:* During a twenty- to thirty-minute workout, vary the intensity every few minutes. Exercise at sixty-five percent of your maximum heart rate for five minutes, then drop down to sixty percent again for the next five minutes. Continue varying your intensity for the whole workout. This will speed up your metabolism.

▸ *Strength Training (Redesigning):* Focus on the chest, shoulders, and arms. The repetitions should be eight to ten per set, with three sets per exercise, per body part. This session should last up to twenty-five minutes.

Since your body is heavy at the hips, thighs, and buttocks then avoid completely any exercises that will bulk the muscles in the lower body. This includes any compound movements such as leg presses, squats, or power dead lifts. Also avoid the stair-climbing machines and high-resistance stationary bike riding. A hip isolation machine is excellent for targeting the hips and buttocks area. Also ride a stationary bike at low resistance. Try isolation movements like high-repetition ninety-degree side leg lifts (hydrants) and iso-lunges.

Bananas

▸ *Aerobic Sessions:* Try walking, stair climbing, or cycling. You will want to keep the intensity low, allowing for a longer session. This aerobic session is done on your "off" days from your body redesigning workouts. Ideally, you should exercise starting at thirty minutes and build up to forty-five minutes. This will assist your body in losing excess body fat.

▸ *Cardiovascular Interval Training Sessions:* During a twenty- to twenty-five-minute workout, vary the intensity every few minutes. Keep the intensity from dropping too low. Exercising at sixty-five percent of your maximum heart rate for five minutes or so and then dropping down to sixty percent for five more is a good mix. This will stimulate your metabolism.

▸ **_Strength Training (Redesigning):_** Because your genetics typically lack curves, building muscle (lean, not bulky) on the upper and lower body works best. Focus equally on the upper and lower body with compound exercises for the lower body such as bench squats, deep-knee bends, or weighted lunges; and weighted exercises for the upper body such as dumbbell chest press, around-the-world for shoulders, and tricep/bicep dumbbell exercises.

Since your body type is such that your upper and lower body are equal or straight up and down, then you are not as concerned with balancing your body's shape as you are to adding curves. By placing emphasis on reducing the waistline, broadening the shoulders and adding curves to your hips, this can be accomplished. See below:

Note: All body types will want to include core work (abdominal exercises) such as reverse crunches, twists, and regular crunches. This session should go for twenty to twenty-five minutes.

Troubleshooting for Best Results

When your automobile is not performing properly the smart thing to do is have a mechanic troubleshoot to find the problem(s). As you plan to redesign your body you, too, must take into account your body's genetic characteristics to discover problem areas so you can know what to do to correct them. The information below includes all three body types, their weight distribution problems, and inherited genetic problems with strategies you can apply to troubleshoot and maximize your results.

Troubleshooting the Pear Body Type

Problem Areas

Weight Distribution Problems

▸ When the pear gains weight, the weight mostly goes to the hips, thighs, and buttocks.

Lower Body

▸ Most body fat accumulates in the hips, thighs, and buttocks.

▸ Considered bottom heavy

Upper Body

▸ Generally slender

▸ Shallow bustline

▸ Narrow shoulders

▸ Straight waist

Inherited Genetic Problems

The following are the primary inherent genetic factors:

▸ Narrow shoulders due to short clavicles

▸ Shallow and small bustline due to less upper body fat

▸ Wide pelvic and hip structure

▸ Excessive adipose fat tissue (cells) on the hips, thighs, and buttocks

▸ Straight waistline due to narrow or small ribs

Body Redesigning Strategies

Perform exercises designed to enhance:

Upper Body

▶ Fill out chest/bust

▶ Broaden back and add width to the shoulders

▶ Firm and tone the arms (biceps and triceps)

▶ Firm the abdominal muscles

Lower Body

▶ Isolate hips, thighs, and buttocks

▶ Elongate, firm, and tone

▶ Reduce lower body major muscles

Avoid any exercises or physical activities that would tend to stimulate the lower body to grow. Concentrate on building muscle mass for the upper body while reducing the lower body.

See: *Fork in the Road*—Body Type DVD/ Pear Workout (Appendix B).

Troubleshooting the Apple Body Type

Problem Areas

Weight Distribution Problems

▶ When the apple gains weight, the weight mostly goes to the upper body. The apple lacks upper body/lower body symmetry or balance.

Lower Body

▶ Generally lagging in size when compared to the upper body

Upper Body

▶ Most body fat stored around the waist, upper back, and arms

Inherited Genetic Problems

The following are the primary inherent genetic factors:

▶ Excessive adipose tissue on the upper body, usually in the abdominal region, the chest/bust, back, and arms
▶ Abdominal muscles usually protrude forward or bulge outward
▶ Generally longer upper torso and shorter lower torso
▶ Thin legs and buttocks, in some instances too thin or undersized from a symmetrical viewpoint

Body Redesigning Strategies

Performing exercises that enhance:

Upper Body

- Shape and tone only
- Isolate abdominal muscles

Lower Body

- Build the upper and lower leg muscles
- Build, firm, and tone the buttocks

Avoid exercises that tend to build mass on the upper body. Exercises for the upper body should be done for the sole purpose of firming and toning each muscle group. Concentrate on the abdominal muscles for strengthening and flattening. Incorporate exercise that will stimulate lower body muscles. Using dumbbells will help develop a symmetrical hourglass shape.

See: *Fork in the Road*—**Body Type DVD/ Apple Workout (Appendix B).**

Troubleshooting the Banana Body Type

Problem Areas

Weight Distribution Problems

When the banana gains weight, the weight goes equally to the upper and lower body.

▶ Mainly lacks curves or shapeliness

▶ Tends to have a straight-line figure or physique

Inherited Genetic Problems

The following are the primary inherent genetic factors:

▶ The musculoskeletal system is such that the pelvic bone, ribs, and shoulder width are similar.

▶ Wide waistline due to above

▶ Adipose fat tissues evenly dispersed on the upper and lower body

Body Redesigning Strategies

Perform exercises that enhance:

Upper Body

▶ Firm, tone, and build muscles; strengthen and tone the abdominal muscles

Lower Body

▸ Elongate the thighs; firm and tone the buttocks

The banana shape may be somewhat confusing to identify. The idea of having a banana shape makes you think the body would be thin. This is true in most cases until the banana gains weight. Then the thin banana becomes a full banana, and the weight is dispersed equally in the upper and lower body. Both banana types (thin and heavy) must incorporate exercises that will even out their shape and add curves and lines. Because the upper and lower body are relatively balanced, or symmetrical, the fuller bananas will want to add additional cardiovascular workouts to their body redesigning program.

See: *Fork in the Road*—Body Type DVD/ Banana Workout (Appendix B).

Having a better understanding of your body type gives you a better understanding of what you have to work with. You will have realistic expectations and can set attainable goals. Regardless of your body type, you have a genetic potential that can be reached. No body type is better than other body types, but each body type requires its own exercise strategy to be *successfully redesigned.*

— Renewing Your Mind —

() Many men and women have desperately tried to reach their body redesigning goals but eventually missed their goal no matter what they did. Has that been your experience? Yes, or no? If yes, then don't feel alone or feel bad about it—most people have. Remember, while it's true that you have to work with what you have, there are some very specific exercises you can do—and others you should avoid—that will help you improve your "body symmetry" and attain the look that your genetics will allow.

() Redesigning your body requires a plan. Are you are ready to redesign your body? I hope your answer is yes. The suggestions in this chapter are definitely a great place to start because they show you how to identify your specific genetic characteristics such as problem areas, inherited genetic problems, and weight distribution problems. Remember: there is not a "best" body type. Every body type has a genetic potential that can be reached. Take advantage of the information in this section. As you become more aware of your individuality, redesigning your body will be a pleasant and rewarding experience.

Epilogue

C AN YOU IMAGINE LIVING IN A WORLD WHERE PEOPLE ARE motivated to help other people be all they can be? A world where people recognize how uniquely different each of us is, and yet be able to appreciate the value and worthiness the other person possesses?

You and I can make that dream world a reality.

As you better understand your own individuality, you become better equipped to reach your fullest potential. Whether you have nearly given up on yourself because of past struggles you have experienced with your weight your entire life, or the repeated feelings of discouragement for not attaining the results you have hoped for, there is still hope.

Your journey is not over yet!

My hope for you after you have finished reading this book is that you are prepared to travel down the road that leads to controlling your weight, being more aware of your triggers, and still be able to win your battle. The knowledge in this book comes from years of seeking and striving, not being willing to settle for mediocre, and never allowing negative obstacles to become permanent roadblocks.

Your past failures, whether being unsuccessful in keeping your weight off, making wrong choices, or falling back to unhealthy thinking, are not permanent imprints of what you are. Consider them the salt to savor your future. Everyone fails at something, sometime, but only those who learn from their failures have hope for the future.

As you begin to apply the strategies from all four sections of this book, your world will never be the same again. You will move outside the box of complacency, frustration, and negativity to new and exciting areas of your life that are full of reward and accomplishments. You will continually grow emotionally. Your attitude will become positive and daring. Your body will take on a new look. You will enjoy the fruits of your labor…for life.

Never Go Back was written to bring you hope and inspiration—not for the next ninety days, but for the rest of your life. The practical insights for understanding why your genetic individuality has been the missing link to your weight loss/weight gain experience will revolutionize your ability to manage your weight and obtain optimum health. Identifying those emotional and food triggers—like potholes that have kept your journey thus far a rocky road—will bring you inner peace and self-confidence.

Take from the book all that you can apply and develop the whole person. Then impart your success, knowledge, and excitement to the next person and be a part of helping them **Never Go Back**.

Then perhaps you and I will be a part of making the dream world a reality.

—Dr. Joe

Appendix A

Dr. Joe offers a wide spectrum of in-depth and exhaustive information in his books on how your genetic individuality (your blood type, diet, and body type for proper exercise know-how) is the missing link in diet and exercise.

▶ *My Body, God's Temple*
▶ *Bloodtypes, Bodytypes and YOU, Revised/Updated*
▶ *Bloodtypes, Bodytypes and YOU*
▶ *Seven Pillars of Health*
▶ *The Answer is in Your Bloodtype*

For maximizing optimum health and bodily function, see Dr. Joe's line of Body Genetics dietary supplements.

Colon Health

1. INNER OUT—14 day Colon Cleansing and Detoxifying System
2. PSYLLIUM—fiber in capsules
3. CAPE ALOE—herbal laxative

Digestion
1. Digestive Enzyme Complex—in capsules

Multiple Vitamins/Minerals
1. AM/PM VITAMINS—multiple vitamin/mineral for blood types O, A, B, and AB.

Minerals
1. ConcenTrace—liquid trace minerals
2. Mega Mineral Complex

Calcium
1. Coral Calcium—marine grade imported from Okinawa, Japan

Protein
1. Protein Shakes—Egg white/Soy Isolate
2. ThinTastic—protein bars

Anti-aging
1. HGH Support—Amino Acid complex
2. DHEA—orchestrate your body's demand for hormones

Meal Replacements
1. Chocolate Meal Replacement Bars
2. Strawberry-Filled Cookies

Fat Burners

1. Energy Booster/Fat Burner capsules
2. Trim—fat burner capsules

Water

1. The "Water Ionizer" Machine—turns tap water into alkaline water.

For more detailed, in-depth product information, please visit our website: **www.bodyredesigning.com** or call **1-800-259-2639**

Appendix B

Fork in the Road:
The Road Map for Redesigning a New You

Fork in the Road is a dynamic motivational DVD series designed to assist the individual who is ready to make healthy lifestyle changes. Professional health and fitness trainer and coach Dr. Joseph Christiano implements three fundamental components: Attitude, Diet, and Exercise for successfully reaching one's fullest potential.

As your life coach and personal trainer, Dr. Joe teaches you how to overcome negative influences, make positive decisions, and rediscover your personal worth by challenging your mental attitude. While developing the correct mental attitude you will learn how to reach your physical genetic potential for weight loss, disease-free living, and maximum health. Dr. Joe teaches how to individualize and be most accurate with food and exercise by factoring in your unique genetic individuality.

"The perfect time to reach your fullest potential starts when you come to a Fork in the Road!"

—Dr. Joe

Fork in the Road Components:

6 DVD Topics:

1. Introduction to Series
2. Redesigning Your Attitude
3. Redesigning Your Diet
4. Redesigning Your Exercise
5. Body Type workout programs w/Dr. Joe (Women)
6. Exercise Technique w/workout charts (Men)

Mapping Journal

This component is an aide for recording thoughts plus answering questions from Dr. Joe's coaching lessons.

Charts

1. Body fat percentage—determine body composition
2. Measurement—monitoring chart for progress

Food Cards

Handy business-sized cards with all food groups based on your blood type.

All 3 categories of food cards:

1. Beneficial, Neutral, and Avoid

Selected Bibliography

Associated Press, "Government Order—Exercise," The Orlando Sentinel, January 26, 2000, A–3.

Blumenkrantz, Michael. "Obesity: The World's Oldest Metabolic Disorder," www.quantumhcp.com/ obesity.htm.

Carrier, Karen M. "Breaking Out of the Dieting Prison," Health and Fitness Idea Source, February 1998, 5.

Christiano, Joseph. Seven Pillars of Health (Lake Mary, FL: Creation House, 2000).

Gittleman, Anne Louise. M.S., with James Templeton and Candace Versace. Your Body Knows Best (New York: Pocket Books, a div. of Simon and Schuster, Inc., 1996).

"Government Order—Exercise," The Orlando Sentinel, January 26, 2000, A–3.

"Hypoglycemia," National Diabetes Information Clearing House, www.niddk.nih.gov/health/diabetes/ pubs/hypo/hypo. htm.

"On Health: Protein and Exercise," Orlando Sentinel.

"Statistics and Research," www.medicalinvestment.com/ quotesandstatistics.html; www.caloriecontrol.org/dietfigs.html; and www.aomc.org/HOD2/ general/weight-DIET.html.

"Statistics Related to Overweight and Obesity," National Institute of Diabetes and Digestive and Kidney Diseases (NIDDK), www.niddk.nih.gov/health/nutrit/pubs/statobes.htm.

Weissberg and Christiano. The Answer is in Your Bloodtype. (further expanded with information from Bio-Foods, Inc., Santa Barbara, California).

Wilkins, Rob and Mike O'Hearn. "Obesity! Public Enemy Number One," Natural Muscle Magazine, January 2000.

www.state.id.us/dhw/hwgd_www/ health/hp/part_2.pdf.

www.weight.com/definition.html.

www.4BetterHealth.com.

www.state.id.us/dhw/hwgd_www/ health/hp/part_2.pdf.

About Dr. Joseph Christiano

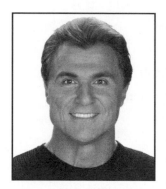 Dr. Joseph Christiano is a naturopathic doctor, certified nutritional counselor, author, motivational speaker, and health and fitness coach. As a guru in the field of body genetic individuality, he specializes in developing customized exercise and nutrition plans. "Dr. Joe," as his friends refer to him, has over 40 years of combined personal and professional experience in the field of health and nutrition. He has redesigned thousands of bodies throughout the world including swimsuit winners in the Miss America and Miss USA pageants, Hollywood stars, and corporate executives, as well as kids from 10 to 70 years of age. His Body Redesigning company, web site, and national seminars have helped thousands of people discover new levels of health and fitness. Also a former body building champion, Dr. Joe works with at-risk kids through his "Dump the Junk" Health and Fitness curriculum and after-school programs. To contact Dr. Joe, email him at drjoe@bodyredesigning.com or go to his Web site at bodyredesigning.com.

About Dwight Bain

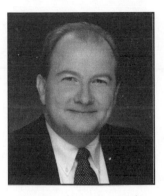 Dwight Bain is a Nationally Certified Counselor & Certified Family Law Mediator. He is an author, speaker, and life coach with a highly successful private practice. Dwight's purpose is to help people achieve maximum results in their personal and professional life. He specializes in helping people manage change, guiding them from stress to success. His insights into "Food Triggers" are heralded by many as ground breaking in the areas of weight management. To contact Dwight Bain go to: www.dwightbain.com